Alive 'n Raw

As Nature Intended

"Eating To Better Health"

Elyse Nuff

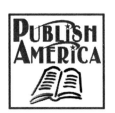

PublishAmerica
Baltimore

First printing

This publication contains the opinions and ideas of its author. Author intends to offer information of a general nature. Neither the author nor the publisher are engaged in rendering medical, health or any other kind of personal professional services to the reader. The reader should consult his or her own physician before relying on any information set forth in or implied from this publication. Any reliance on the information herein is at the reader's own discretion.

The author and publisher specifically disclaim all responsibility for any liability, loss, or right, personal or otherwise, which is incurred as a consequence, directly or indirectly, of the use and application of any contents of this book. They further make no representations or warranties with respect to the accuracy or completeness of the contents of this work and specifically disclaim all warranties including without limitation any implied warranty of fitness for a particular purpose. Any recommendations are made without any guarantee on the part of the author or the publisher.

PublishAmerica has allowed this work to remain exactly as the author intended, verbatim, without editorial input.

Hardcover 978-1-4512-0507-7
Softcover 978-1-4512-0492-6
PUBLISHED BY PUBLISHAMERICA, LLLP
www.publishamerica.com
Baltimore

Printed in the United States of America

Dedication

This book is dedicated to all the people who have the courage to be different and realize that their health is of foremost importance in their lives. You have no greater asset.

It is also dedicated to all my friends who inspired me to be who I am. Thank you.

Thank you to Carole Ann for making sure all my words made sense. Without you, I would be still wondering.

Also a big Thank you to Mary Katherine for her apt assistance in editing this book for me.

Contents

Foreword

Health problems are on the increase today as never before. This is very upsetting but most people just seem to accept the various disease conditions as part of growing older. Obviously, conventional medicine does not have the answers or we would be healthier as a nation. We are not. Disease is not normal! Nor is it natural.

Your body was so wonderfully designed to live trouble-free for a very long time-and to self correct when physical problems arise. However, it needs proper nutrition to do its job. It needs the right tools. Here is the secret— "It takes life to get life." That is where raw food comes in because once food is cooked it becomes dead. It loses the live enzymes and electricity that provide the rejuvenating power for health. Cooked food fills the stomach but it doesn't supply the building blocks your body needs for health.

Furthermore, it costs the body energy and minerals to process it. Over time, this leads to deficiencies and eventual degenerative diseases.

This book *Alive 'n Raw* presents a solution for restoring life back to the body. It points us back to eating the way 'nature intended.' On your search for more energy and renewed health, increasing the amount of good quality raw food in your diet is # 1.

Eating raw food doesn't have to be boring either. Try out the various suggestions and recipes in this book and experiment. After a while, your tastes will change and your body will love you for it. Your body is always looking for a live energy charge. That can only come from raw food.

Ron Garner,
Author of *"After the Doctors"…What Can you Do?" and "The 4 Keys To a Long Life"*

Introduction

During my education and practice as a complementary health practitioner, assisting people back to their own good health, I have discovered that working with herbs alone to clean and rebuild the body is not the total answer. I began to look further into using raw foods together with the herbs to clean up some of the diseases that were plaguing people. The diseases were cleaning up faster and easier when combining the two methods of healing.

The more raw food juices and whole foods that were introduced, the faster and better people were healing. This outcome resulted in more research into why raw foods were such a benefit to people and why they were speeding up the process of healing.

Studies showed that all the nutrients the body requires is already in these raw foods; therefore it only made common sense to me that these were the things lacking in our diets. Further examination showed that heating foods past a certain temperature killed all the live enzymes in foods that we are eating today. We are actually giving our bodies nothing but cooked mush.

My experience now shows me that consuming raw foods with a good, gentle bowel cleanser, will not only assure you of good health but is one of the best weight control plans in the world.

In looking for that "Fountain of Youth," or "Ultimate Health &Vitality," finding it is through adopting a simple back-to-nature diet or lifestyle.

Within these pages is the key to delaying the aging process. We hope you will make use of this book to open up your own experiences and lead a more fulfilling and satisfying life.

Use it as both reference book and recipe book when you are preparing meals for you and your loved ones. This book is dedicated to you and your journey to new and better health through a lifestyle that is unique and very real. As Nature Intended!

For your convenience, I have listed WebPages and Internet sites as reference points for some of the included research in the book and for your further study.

Beginning

Raw foods are fantastic. Known as Nature's own nutrient packed body builders, cleaners, and tonics, they cannot be beaten. The greatest benefit to our bodies is combining them with regular exercise.

Most of us have the potential to have long, healthy lives. Why do we fall short of this goal? Mostly, because we believe that age is creeping up on us, so therefore, we become helpless and sickly as soon as we reach a certain birth-date.

Though we see other people our age who are healthy and vibrant, we don't tend to believe that it can happen to us. It is important to have that belief system working for us. What we believe is what we are, or what we become. (That's a whole new book).

It is our birthright to be healthy and vital all our lives.

Another reason for us falling short of maintaining our good health is our lack of consistency. By not adopting a life-long habit of wholesome eating and regular exercise, we do little to nourish our good health and long life.

It is not what we occasionally eat or drink, nor is it that we do what we should for a short while, then quit, it is our daily intake of nourishing foods that give us our vitality and wholesome life.

That is why it is of vital importance that we choose the freshest, most wholesome raw foods that we can find. Organic and local grown is always best.

Also of vital importance is good, clean, fresh water to wash our food with and to use in our recipes, as well as drink.

These foods, fresh water, and keeping active every day will keep us healthy and strong.

The new venture to Raw Foods can be your first step back in your journey to this healthy and vital life.

I hope this book will help you take that first step, whether you are fighting some disease, or just wanting to be the healthiest you can possibly be.

It may just change your life.

Whatever brings you to this raw living food decision was probably the best reason in the world.

You no doubt have come to realize that you desire a change in your lifestyle. Do you feel as alive as you would like to?

This raw foodism, if you like, gives you an opportunity to be now in control of your own health and your environment.

If you are reading this book, you have started in the right place; we will try to help you make the transition needed to go through, to get there.

The first thing you need to do, is realize and admit that all of the cooked food you have been eating for the past years has become an addiction.

Glitzy advertising and flavours we have come to enjoy actually enslave us. You must be willing to relegate these old habits to oblivion. Don't despair; it is not as hard as you may think it is. We take one step at a time.

An important aspect in adopting this new lifestyle is the willingness to take responsibility for your health and well-being.

This is a "biggy." Many of us are so tied into everything around us, no matter whether it is good or bad for us, we will still do it. Often it is because someone else is doing it, or they are teasing us for not being like them.

Your routine will include changing your eating habits to provide optimal nourishment for your body. If you are willing to change your habits, the aging and disease in your body will be stopped and the process of rejuvenation begun, regardless of your age.

People as old as seventy, eighty, even ninety, can live their most fulfilling and productive years once their lifestyle changes are made.

One of the important essentials is that you eat for nourishment by choosing and preparing foods that render them the most easily digested. No less of importance is the maintaining of a clean colon.

This helps to move out the old toxins and helps the body to rejuvenate. It is also extremely beneficial to have a daily exercise routine of some sort (depending on your daily schedule).You should be able to set up several minutes of exercise a couple of times a day, in order to keep the body moving.

The body is made to be active, and if this is not happening, then the body will become rigid and disease oriented.

Exercise is a big factor in keeping our bodies healthy. There are many ways to do this: walking, using a small rebounder, and taking stairs instead of elevators.

These activities are great for the cardiovascular system and become necessary for the body to detoxify and heal well.

You are working on total body health, not just detoxifying.

No matter what your activity may be, it will contribute to your body's total well being and assist in removing the toxins from your system.

Preparation

Now that you have decided that raw food is for you, you should know that raw food contains all the nutrients your body needs. Yes, even protein, calcium, and all the other minerals and vitamins that are cooked out of foods when you heat them.

Your raw food adventure starts in the kitchen. Here is a list of some of the implements you will need to prepare your meals. You life will become simplified and easy. Here they are:

Blender
Cutting Board
Dehydrator
Food Processor
Grater
Juicer
Nut chopper
Potato Peeler

These tools will make your food preparation much simpler. Don't panic if you don't have something; plan to acquire it for a special occasion or event. You also do not have to have the fanciest or costliest equipment advertised. Just acquire what you can get and they will work just as well.

Foods and Their NutrientContent

Following is a list detailing some of the minerals etc. that will help guide you in your choices of food. Always buy **ORGANIC** foods whenever possible. They have no herbicides or pesticides. The organic soil is not depleted of nutrients and is replenished in the proper manner to retain these nutrients. Therefore, the foods coming from it are also very rich in nutrients.

I cannot list all the foods here, as there are hundreds, but following are some of the most well-known foods, and their nutrient value.

Protein: avocado, nuts, seeds, sea veggies

Fiber: avocado, figs, guava, prunes, pumpkin, sea veggies, blueberries, cabbage family, cantaloupe, cauliflower, carrots, cherries, currants, cranberries

Calcium: pineapple, carrot, cherry, grapefruit, pear, raspberry, beet greens, blueberry, broccoli, sea veggies, dark leafy greens

Selenium: carrot, sea vegetables, garlic, Red Swiss Chard,

Potassium: pineapple, apricot, carrot, cherry, grapefruit, grapes, mango, orange, passion fruit, paw paw, peaches, pears, watermelon pumpkin, beets & greens, broccoli, cantaloupe, cranberries, guava, okra, banana, avocado, most fresh veggies, onion, prunes, and pumpkin

Anti-Oxidants: blueberries (increase intake), carrots, all red, or yellow foods, sea vegetables, watermelon, beets & greens, sweet potato

Sulphur: pineapple, garlic, onion

Iron: pineapple, apple, apricot, parsley, and sea vegetables

Omega-3 Fats: avocado, nuts, seeds, flax seeds & oil, olive oil, walnuts

Zinc: orange, pumpkin seeds, ginger root, pecans, and brazil nuts

Manganese: grapes, melon, nuts, okra, spinach

Copper: apricot, seeds, brazil nuts, almonds, hazelnuts, and pecans

Iodine: pineapple, melon, sea salt, sea vegetables, spinach, and kelp

Sodium: celery, sea salt, carrot, and pineapple.

Magnesium: apple, apricot, dark leafy greens, cherry, nuts, raspberry, and beet greens

Phosphorous: carrot, grapefruit, orange, pears, pineapple, grapes, okra, pumpkin, sea veggies, spinach, kiwi, passion fruit

B Vitamins: paw paw, pear, peach, apricot, carrot, grapes, lemon, mango, raspberry, nuts, banana, green tea, onions, dark leafy greens, watermelon, cherry, spinach

B12: dulse, bean sprouts

A Vitamins: watermelon, apricot, carrot, pineapple, banana, broccoli, pumpkin, cherry, spinach, sweet potato, melon, peaches, pears

C Vitamins apple, apricot, blackberry, carrot, cherry, grapefruit, grapes, passion fruit, pineapple, raspberry, kiwi, lemon, avocado, blueberry, mango, orange, paw paw, pears, broccoli, cabbage family, cantaloupe, cauliflower, chili peppers, cranberries, onion, spinach, sweet potato, watermelon, brussel sprouts, turnip, dark green leafy veggies, black current, green tea, guava,

E Vitamins: carrot, walnuts, seeds

D Vitamins: morning sunshine, at least 10-15 minutes daily.

Folic Acid: seeds, carrot, parsley, spinach, sweet potato, watermelon, pears, apricot, broccoli, cantaloupe, cauliflower, okra, nuts, cherry, grapefruit, beet greens, grapes, melon, dark leafy greens

K Vitamins: dark leafy greens, cruciferous veggies, okra, cauliflower, spinach

Minerals/Trace: pineapple, figs, apple, nuts, legumes, dark leafy greens, apricot, cherry, carrot,, pineapple, grapefruit, lemon, orange, parsley

Cooked
Food

Many raw food advocates actually believe that one should begin slowly and progress to a 100% raw food diet. Personal experience shows that this method only tends to prolong your cooked food cravings and slows down the healing process in your body.

If this is not a possibility for you, then you should definitely take it slowly, and gradually work up to the 100% diet, instead of not doing it at all. The more raw food you can incorporate into your diet the more chances of your health improving.

Again, my research is that, if you want to embrace this lifestyle for optimum health reasons, go 100% raw, and deal with the cravings you may experience with a raw food replacement (some helpful replacements in a later chapter).

The very first thing we must address is that we are addicted to the cooked food lifestyle. Yummy. It tastes and looks so good. Get that smell into your nostrils. Look at that ad in the newspaper or on the television of people digging in to eat with gusto. No ad will ever begin to hint that this cooked food is poison to your body… yes poison.

The body cannot digest this food, as it is a dead food. The body can only digest live nutrition; it builds up a layer of mucus to protect itself, and soon distributes it through your system as a plug.

Therefore, no nutrients can get to your organs and glands, etc. Your body needs 123 nutrients and over 2,000 trace minerals for you to be alive.

Cooking the food you eat destroys all the nutrients it possesses when reaching over 105 degrees F. That's not very high, so cooking is destruction.

Cooked food clogs the capillaries that are between every cell in your body. Some symptoms of this clogging are: sore legs, weak legs, exhaustion, and lethargy, tired all the time. Usually the sore, weak legs first warn you of something amiss.

That is because the circulation is slower to the lower portions of the body and it is more difficult to return the blood up to the heart, and the cooked food is making the blood clump, clog, and run slower still.

Upon study of an actual microscopic view of the blood after eating both raw and cooked food, it is amazing what happens. On raw food the person's blood stream is clear and very active, alive, no sludge to be seen. When cooked food is introduced to this same body, the blood stream was clogged, sticky and hardly moving, with a cloudy look to it. In addition, this took place within 7 hours of this person eating cooked food.

Did you know that the body actually sets up a layer of mucus in your stomach to protect you from the poisons of the cooked food going into your blood stream and killing you? When you eat salad greens and raw fruits & veggies along with your cooked food meal, most of the nutrients are lost to your body because of this layer of mucus, as the mucus blocks them from being distributed throughout the body.

The body cannot digest this food, so it is therefore pushed through and discarded as feces.

The mucus then settles into the bottom of our lungs, allowing it to be expelled when we become active. If this does not happen, the mucus keeps building up in our lungs and then into other areas of the body, even the brain, causing muddled thinking and sluggishness.

Cooked food is poison

What does your blood look like today? Do you feel sluggish? Are you low on energy? After you eat, do you feel like a nap? Cooked food is poison. Ever wonder why you have to clear your throat more often, these days? Ahhem…….

You can change that.

Raw food is living. Your body is living, rejuvenating all the time.

Did you know that it only takes six weeks for your liver to be totally new again? Your skin renews in 3-4 weeks. You have a completely new stomach lining in only 4 days. In addition, your eyes have completely replicated in only 2 days.

It is amazing how our bodies are able to be very new in such short times. We must be willing to assist these changes in any way we can. Raw food is giving the body all the help it needs, to keep you renewed and healthy.

Therefore, I applaud your raw food lifestyle change, and congratulate you on your decision. You have made a wise choice.

The road may not be easy, but then who ever said being different and healthy is easy?

You can make this change easier on yourself by accepting comments about this change and suggesting that you are doing this 'for your health.'

The hardest part of your transition to raw food will be staying away from the temptations.

The cooked food will smell and look very good for about the first two months. You must be prepared to abstain and have a plan to refuse the cooked food and not upset anyone by doing so.

Not everyone will understand why you are doing this and some will get on your case. One way to help yourself is to bring a dish you would like to eat along with you. People are happy to have you do this and it more or less takes them off the hook as to what you would eat at a dinner party.

This takes the tension away from the scene and allows everyone to be comfortable with your new diet. Having a dish that can include the rest of the table also helps them realize you are not just eating "rabbit food."

These measures make the transition much easier and help you stick by your decision to stay raw "for your health."

Let other people continue to eat whatever they choose, and gradually they will see how well you are doing and witness the positive changes that are happening within you. You will become a shining example. They will see your energy, stamina, and glowing health and will want to become like that themselves.

It's easier to change someone's religion than the way they eat.

Why Eat Raw

Clearly, your diet is the basis for good health and optimum healing. Recent research on nutraceuticals and phytonutrients in our food provides a wealth of evidence to support the fact that our diets can heal as well as nourish us.

Diet improvement is a major weapon against disease; from the common cold to cancer.

Whole, raw food nutrition allows the body to use its built-in restorative and repairing abilities. A healthy diet can intervene in the disease process at many stages, from its inception to its growth and spread. Fresh fruits and vegetables top the list of healing foods.

Massive research is validating what natural healers have known for decades. The more fruits and vegetables you eat, the more nutrition you get and the less risk of disease.

Raw fresh fruits and vegetables do what natural healers do best…work with your body so it can use its built-in restorative abilities.

Even if your DNA and lifestyle are against you, your diet still makes a tremendous difference in your health and healing odds.

Raw fresh fruits and vegetables accelerate body cleansing, and help normalize body chemistry. Raw fruits and vegetables are full of nutraceuticals, the natural chemicals in plants and have pharmacological action. Scientists are enthusiastically embracing the healing possibilities of plant nutrients in fresh foods.

Green leafy vegetables, for example, have almost 20 times more essential nutrients, ounce for ounce, than any other food.

What is more, the nutrients in greens make the nutrients in other foods work better towards our health. The preventive medicine possibilities are astounding. Studies show that people who eat plenty of vegetables have half the cancer risk than do people who eat few raw vegetables.

Certain body chemicals must be "activated" before they initiate cancer cell growth. Raw fresh foods can block that activation process, because food chemicals in cells can determine whether a cancer-causing virus or a cancer promoter, such as excess estrogen will turn tissue cancerous. Raw fruits and vegetables may intervene even if you already have cancer.

When cells mass into tumors, the food compounds in cruciferous vegetables can retrain further growth by flushing certain carcinogens from the body, or by shrinking patches of precancerous cells. Antioxidant foods can snuff out carcinogens, nip free radical cascades in the bud, and even repair some cellular damage.

New studies on fruits show benefits that are even more amazing. Citrus fruits possess fifty-eight known anti-cancer compounds, more than any other food.

Some researchers call citrus fruits a total anti-cancer package because they have every class of nutrient-carotenoids, flavonoids, terpens, limonoids, coumarins, and more—known to neutralize chemical carcinogens.

Citrus fruits act more powerfully, as a whole, than any of the separate anti cancer compounds they contain.

One phytochemical, for example found in orange juice, unlike in whole oranges, loses its glutathione concentration when juiced. Oranges are also rich in beta-carotene and Vitamin C, and are the highest food in glucarate, a powerful cancer-inhibitor.

Raw, green leafy vegetables exhibit extraordinary broad cancer protective power largely because they are so rich in antioxidants. Alpha, beta, and other carotenes, folic acid and zeaxanthin in greens offer potent cancer protection. The darker green in colour the vegetable is, the more cancer-inhibiting carotenoids they have. This also gives you an extraordinary amount of enzymes, which your body needs to function.

Enzymes are your life spark and help the body to distribute calcium to your bones, and help make your blood function properly. If you do not replenish your enzymes daily, they will become depleted and you die. Enzymes are a most important part of your diet.

Your raw green leafy vegetables are the best source of these enzymes. That is why we recommend a green leafy salad each day.

They are the cornerstones of healing because they are the foundation elements of the immune system, providing active antioxidants that fight free-radical destruction.

Enzymes operate at both chemical and biological levels.

Chemically, they are the workhorses that drive metabolism to use the nutrients that we take in. Biologically, they are our life energy. Without enzyme energy, we would be a pile of lifeless chemicals.

Each of us is born with a battery charge of enzyme energy at birth. As we age, our internal enzyme stores are naturally depleted. Enzyme depletion, lack of energy, disease, and aging, all go hand in hand. Unless we stop the one-way flow out of our bodies of enzyme energy, our digestive-elimination capabilities weaken, obesity and chronic illness sets in, and life span shortens.

The faster we use up our enzymes supply-the shorter our life span.

Raw plant enzymes offer built-in enzyme therapy. They give the body what it needs to work properly.

Our body chemistry comes from plant nutrients because plant chlorophyll transmits the energies of the sun and the soil to our bodies. The sun is the energy source of the Earth—plants constitute the most direct method of conserving the energy we receive from the sun.

Raw fruits, vegetables, and grasses reach out to us on branches and stems, making themselves beautiful and nourishing to attract us. Plants have no fear of being eaten as animals do.

The life energy of plants simply transmutes into the higher life form of humankind. This takes us to the importance of the enzyme replacement each day by raw fruits and vegetables.

Be aware that some people start craving raw food, because they come to love the taste of it. They then come to crave this more than they did the cooked food they used to eat.

And God said; Behold, I have given you every herb bearing seed, which is upon the face of the earth, and every tree, in which is the fruit of a tree yielding seed; to you it shall be for meat…Genesis 1:29

Why Detoxification

Detoxification means different things to different people. Some say they cannot live without it, others don't know what it is. A lot of cultures fast on a regular basis to initiate detoxification of the body.

This fasting is done by taking only water for one or more days a week to assist their lymphatics to remove the wastes that have accumulated in their tissues. They understand that the build up of toxins in the body causes all kinds of diseases.

Today, there is more consideration given to the fact that our whole system is affected by the toxins in our body. We now know that they affect our physical, mental and emotional beings.

A lot of the cancer is caused by the air we breathe, the food we eat, and the water we drink.

Over the last eighty years all degenerative diseases have increased dramatically, such as heart disease, diabetes, cancer, cystic fibrosis, arthritis, emphysema, multiple sclerosis, chronic fatigue, AIDS, etc. These diseases are more rampant because we are exposed to more toxins today than ever before.

The oils, water, and vegetables that our body needs for self-cleaning and rebuilding of the body have all become carriers of the poisons we are exposed to today. No wonder our systems are burdened with toxins and overrun with diseases.

It isn't a matter of curing the disease, it is a matter of removing these toxins from the body before they cause a disease.

Organic foods are now giving us the tools to have a healthy, vital lifestyle again, without toxins.

Detoxification begins in the bowel (large intestine or colon), as it is the waste removal system of the body. The waste materials from the foods we eat are dispersed through the bowel to clean the system.

When this system is not functioning properly, the waste material does not leave the body properly and will begin to cause problems.

According to the Chinese, the bowel is the most important of the body's organs and glands, and they consider it to be the cause of all diseases.

This is where we begin our journey to good health.

Before, or as you are starting any health regime, it is recommended that one should clean the bowel.

It is imperative that one finds out how the bowel eliminates and how this affects your health. Why would one do this, you might ask, thinking that one's bowel is working just fine.

The first reason may be that a person wants to see the results happening, from whatever regime one is working with, to better their health.

Secondly, a clean bowel is the only way the live nutrients can get into the rest of the organs and glands to feed the body.

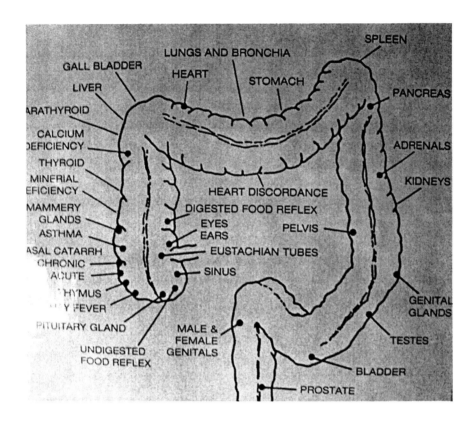

This bowel feeds all the organs and glands the nutrition from the food we eat, it is clean and functioning properly. This bowel is healthy. It doesn't need any help. It is helping the body.

It is now known that nearly every person living in today's society is constipated. Even though the bowel may move every day, people are still constipated.

This means that the feces are impacted together within the bowel and old, hardened feces are sticking to the walls of the bowel, not being eliminated with the regular bowel movements. This constipation is so prominent today that everyone considers it to be natural, even traditional medicine.

Few people really know how much of this hardened fecal matter they are carrying around in their bodies every day. You could be carrying up to 25-30 lbs. of this matter in your body right now.

The hardened feces are formed from the liquid, slimy matter that is passing through your bowel. If it moves slower, it will lose more of its moisture during this passage, and will become more compacted within the bowel. It becomes sticky and glues a coat of itself to the walls of the bowel as it passes through.

Over time, these layers of gluey feces are attached to the walls of the bowel and become hardened into a rubbery-like black substance.

These feces may gather in pockets in your bowel or attach themselves to the full length of the bowel walls, and sometimes move up into the small intestine.

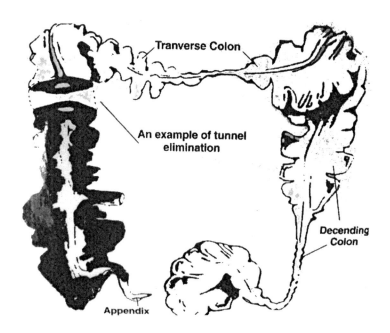

This bowel has the black, gluey, feces sticking to the inside walls of it. Plus, it has diverticuli as well, which is hard, rotting and not moving. This bowel is feeding the body toxins. This bowel is in trouble. This bowel needs help.

In today's society, there are so many mucus and toxic forming substances that help to form these hardened feces. Many of these stagnant feces have been in the bowel for a lifetime. This concentration of toxic, hard substances in the bowel can raise havoc in the rest of the body as well as the bowel.

These toxins, released by the decaying process, harbor a large amount of harmful bacteria and become released into the bloodstream and the organs and glands, traveling to all parts of the body. Every cell in the body becomes affected and it weakens the entire system. This putrefaction should never be allowed to happen.

This bowel should be eliminating at least twice daily. It is meant to hold only one meal at a time.

That means one meal in and one meal out. That is the way the system is made to work. We see very little of this happening today. What is happening to the other bowel movements that are not happening each day? They are becoming putrefacted in the bowel.

This according to the Chinese can be the cause of the diseases of the body in our society today. You will never attain good health again, until these old, hardened feces are removed from your body.

These feces do not pass out of the body during regular bowel movements. They require special techniques to dissolve and remove them from the bowel walls.

The ordinary laxative does not loosen these feces, so therefore something more softening and dissolving is needed to have them removed gently from the bowel walls and out of the bowel.

This colon cleansing, as it is called, is the key, to have not only the bowel become clean again, but is an advantage to the whole body health.

Being that the bowel feeds the nutrients to the rest of the organs and glands in the body, a clogged bowel cannot do this.

The live raw nutrients will just pass right through the bowel without being utilized by the system. Therefore you are losing the benefits of all the vitamins, minerals, amino acids, etc. that the body needs to be healthy. Remember, these live raw nutrients are being fed to the organs and glands through the bowel as they are worked through to elimination.

As a result, you may think that to take replacement supplements for this lack of nutrition, or to heal the issue in your body, is the answer to the problem. The body is not in an optimum state to use these supplements and they are passing through your body and bowel without being of any benefit to your system. The hard feces in your bowel are blocking this passage as it did to the raw live nutrients.

Therefore this is another reason why the bowel needs to be cleansed of the old feces, and give your body and bowel the health it deserves.

Everyone should start their health regime, or the introduction of raw foods to their diets, with at least two months of using a good, softening, bowel cleanser, to eliminate these problems, and allow the bowel to begin functioning properly and on its own again. (My bowel cleanser recommendation can be found at: http://www.LiveRawKitchen.com/bowel.php click on herbal products.)

You will experience the absorption of the raw live nutrients to your system and your energy, stamina and clarity will change dramatically. You will be absorbing the vitamins, nutrients, amino acids, etc. that your body requires to be healthy and vital.

When the bowel is healthy, the body is healthy.

Why
Fasting

Before starting your raw food diet, one should learn the art of fasting. Fasting also helps the bowel and body to continue to cleanse, after the old feces have been removed from the bowel.

What is Fasting you say?

NOT EATING! Just drink water. This could be done one day before you start your raw food diet. It will help the cleansing start to take place. It is one of the most beneficial things you will do for your body.

Fasting and living the raw food diet should go hand in hand. Fasting should be an important part of any raw food regime, to help your body rest from digesting food, and direct its attention to cleaning it.

A bowel cleanser should be used while fasting to keep the toxins moving from your system, as the toxins are dumped into your colon when cleaned from other parts of your body.

It is important to keep them moving out of your system. As you are not eating any solid foods during your fast, the colon will slow down and not eliminate.

This allows the toxins to be reabsorbed, if they are not leaving the body.(For further interest of body cleansers please see http://www.simplylivingsuperfoods.com.com)

You come off a fast by drinking fruit juices, then salads, and then finally you can start on the heavier foods like shredded vegetables, nut loaves, and pates.

You may continue to do this once a week, ideally the same day each week, choosing a day convenient for you not to eat, just drink water.

As you progress in your raw food lifestyle, you may want to fast longer periods to help your body.

This will help give your body its optimum health. Fasting up to a week or ten days has helped others to gain better health.

Don't stress it, do what your body indicates to you it may need, and follow its guidelines.

You may expect some other changes in your body as you are detoxifying. Some of them may be: weakness, fatigue, headaches, swelling in the legs or lower extremities, flu symptoms, rashes, symptoms of old viruses still left in the body and detoxifying through the pores. None of these events are reason for concern.

This is part of the cleaning process your body is going through. Welcome them, as you are getting better.

It is always a good idea to rest your body as much as you can when it is going through the cleaning process, as the body needs the energy to clean.

You do not want to take this energy away from it by being active. This time will benefit the body greatly in its cleaning process.

If one is experiencing fever or flu symptoms, do not take medication for relief to settle it down. The body will then turn its attention from cleaning your body of the fever, and try to get rid of the chemical toxin you put into your body.

A fever is a good sign from the body. It can indicate the body is eradicating some heavy toxins from itself. Welcome it; it usually only lasts about 36 hours.

Having a high fever is not dangerous. It is your body letting you know it is doing its job. That is why a fever goes away when you take something for it.

It isn't because the chemical took the fever away, but because the body switched its job. It was more important to get the chemical out of your body first.

Always rest when you have a fever and assist the body in its work. The best way to assist is to drink lots of clean pure water.

As you begin your new lifestyle, you will notice your body going through some other changes as well. You will begin to lose weight. DON'T PANIC!

This is natural for your body to do, as your body is now shedding all the old, bad fat that has been accumulating in your body over your lifetime.

Lean, strong, truly healthy cells and muscles will replace this. This will not happen all at once. It will take awhile as you detoxify. Continuing with your new lifestyle, you will begin to gain GOOD fat and weight back again.

Why
Live
Enzymes

Enzymes are so important to your health that they deserve a chapter of their own. Enzymes are your life force. You must have enzymes in your body to live. They are your "spark of life." If your enzymes are depleted, you die.

At birth, we are given a reserve of enzymes. Without replacing these enzymes with live, nutritious enzymes, they become depleted. The body can only use the live enzymes for refueling.

If there is disease present in the body, one must look to the enzyme level in the body, as this is usually where the problem is occurring.

If the enzyme level is low, disease is present. There is no disease that can survive in the body if our enzyme bank is complete and functioning properly.

A person does not become ill if this enzyme bank is full and the enzymes are successful in removing the cause of the disease and maintaining the body in good health.

Enzymes are the life and healing force within the body, states the book "*After the Doctors…What Can You Do?, written by Ron Garner.*

Enzymes assist the body in repairing itself. For instance, if a bone is broken in the body, enzymes help the calcium to be absorbed by that bone, to help it to heal. Enzymes support all types of healing in the body. Enzymes assist in the digestion of foods in the body. If there is a lack of enzymes, age and disease creeps into the body and the body begins to deteriorate. This is losing your enzyme "spark."

There are many different kinds of enzymes in the body and they are only replaced with live enzymes from raw live foods. There are three forms of enzymes found in the body.

There are food enzymes, which are replaced with raw live foods, such as organic fruits, vegetables, nuts and seeds: digestive enzymes, which are put out by the pancreas, stomach and small intestine: and metabolic enzymes that are put out by the body to run the metabolic processes.

Did you know that every second in the body, there are multitudes of cells being renewed or created within the body?

Each cell requires millions of specific biochemical steps that are triggered and accelerated by enzymes in the body? Some of the renewals take place quickly: a completely new stomach lining in 4 days, new liver cells in 4-6 weeks, new eye cells in 2 days. You would have a completely new cell system within seven months to one year.

Live raw food sources are the only source of enzymes your body can use to help rebuild these cells.

These enzymes are lost when foods we eat are heated over 105 degrees F.

Other ways these enzymes are lost are by using chemicals, radiation, exposure to oxygen and fluoridation. *Fluoride is one *See: Appendix F of the most dangerous poisons in our society. It is 15 times more poisonous than arsenic.

Pasteurization is another way the enzymes are taken from our foods, as it heats the products until the enzyme activity is gone. Other ways of losing enzymes from the body include nicotine and caffeine. They destroy multitudes of enzymes each time they are put into the body.

When we do not get adequate enzymes from our foods, the body must manufacture them, using the enzymes from its own bank of enzymes in order to do this. This in time depletes the bank of enzymes and wears the body down, and disease and aging starts taking place in the body.

Because of this, it is easy to understand that by eating cooked and processed foods, the body becomes short of enzymes, acidic and disease sets in.

Enzymes also need the help of vitamins, minerals and oils to work properly within the body.

The body works as a team. No one part works properly without another part. This also holds true for the enzyme activity within our body. When our food is not supplying the proper nutrients for this activity, it leads to shortage of reserves and diseases set into the body.

To defend itself from the cooked food we put into the body, the body forms a layer of mucus to protect our blood from receiving the poisons from the lifeless food. The digestion of this food becomes nearly impossible as the body considers it to be dead and poisonous to the body.

This results in a high count of white blood cells as well, because of the lack of enzymes in the cooked food being given to the body. These white blood cells are trying to clear the body of the toxins created by this dead food. In an effort to create more enzymes to try and digest this food, it becomes weaker and more disease ridden, over time.

Remember, enzyme resources directly attribute to the body's energy, strength and health.

When enzymes are low, so are the activities, functioning and metabolic functions of the whole body.

Also, the quantity of enzymes the body has is a measure of its vitality and life.

Fortunately, we have good, organic, raw, live foods to replenish our body each and every day.

"We already have the precious mixture that will make you well, use it"…Rumi

Why
Water

*Water is very important to your system. If you do not have water your system dehydrates and soon breaks down. Water is the second most important thing to your body, next to oxygen. Your body is made up of 67% water, therefore it is vital for the cells. They rely on it to function properly, keep them working and able to replicate properly.

Even your brain needs water to keep the messages in your brain cells that travel on "water-ways" traveling into your nerve endings. Water also transports all the minerals, vitamins and nutrients throughout your body for assimilation. Water keeps you cool and keeps you in balance, moistens your tissues and flushes away your toxins.

Enough water will give your skin hydration, and gives your joints, bones and muscles fluid as shock absorbers. Water even adds minerals to your body.

*See: Appendix F

Your body works at its peak when it gets enough water.

Water helps the body's functions, such as fluid retention decreases, glands and hormone functions improve, the liver functions better thus releasing more fat, even hunger is curtailed when you are not dehydrated.

By the time you want a drink, you are already greatly dehydrated. Dehydration plays a big roll in the body becoming constipated, bladder and kidney infections happen, problems like hemorrhoids and varicose veins become part of your life. It even plays a part in arthritis in your body.

When you reduce the intake of fats into your diet (including omega 3 and other essential fatty acids), the body does not hold and use the water you do take in.

This is one reason that sea greens are recommended to be included in your diet. They help you to have moister skin, shining eyes and lustrous hair. Oils such as flax seed oil, hemp oil, olive oil and nuts are essential benefits to your water intake.

Water quality is poor in most areas of the world today. Most tap water is chlorinated and/or fluoridated, so much so that it can be irritating to the body instead of a nourishing drink. There arc over 500 different disease causing bacteria, viruses and parasites in our waters today.

*Fluoridated water increases the absorption of such things as aluminum from foil wrap, pots, pans, and other dishes or containers used. This is a possible concern for aging quicker, as well as the possibility of causing brain Dementia or Alzheimer's Disease.

Chemicals used by industry and agriculture are also a concern, as they become lodged in our ground water, adding many more pollutants.

The body exerts itself to dispose of these heavy chemicals.

*See: Appendix F

Not having this body effort working for you, you would have ingested enough of these toxins in a lifetime to turn you into stone.

This keeps many people from using tap water. Get yourself a Brita filter and/or a filter on your fridge and keep those heavy toxins from being in your drinking water and having it drinkable and beneficial to your body.

All you need to do is drink more water! Here's how the body uses it up EVERY DAY.

Your kidneys receive and filter the entire body supply 15 times each hour! If you become overheated, your 2 million sweat glands are using 99% of your water to perspire, to cool the skin and the internal organs, keeping them at a constant temperature. You use a small amount of water during blinking your eyelids, 25 times per minute.

Sneezing and heavy breathing release water from the eyes and nose. Even normal activity uses up a least 3 quarts of replacement water each day. Strenuous activity, a hot climate, or high table salt diet increases this requirement.

What happens when you don't get enough water? A chain reaction begins:

1. A water shortage message is sent from the brain.

2. The kidneys conserve water by urinating less (constipation and bloating occur).

3. At 4% water depletion, muscle endurance diminishes—you start to get lethargic.

4. At 5% water loss, headaches from mild to quite severe begin— you become drowsy, lose the ability to concentrate, and become unreasonably impatient.

5. At 6% water loss, body temperature is impaired, and the heart begins to race.

5. At 7% body water depletion, there is a good possibility of collapse.

To check whether or not you are drinking enough water, check your urine. The colour should be pale straw and you should urinate every few hours. If the urine is dark yellow, start drinking more WATER!

You should drink 1/2 the body weight of water in ounces daily. Example: 180 lbs = 90 ounces of water daily. Use 1/8 tsp. of Celtic Sea Salt to every quart of water you drink. As long as you drink the water you can have Celtic Sea Salt.

Oils
And
Fats

We must understand that the body needs oils from our diet. The body cannot make the essential fatty acids contained in good oils. Staying on a low-fat diet long enough leads to disease and death.

Being aware of the difference between the good oils and the bad fats is our responsibility.

The body does not know the difference. The body cannot use the bad fats we give it.

The essential oils (fatty acids) are used by the body to rebuild cell structure, transport nutrients, and to produce hormones. These oils are needed to produce energy and for the functioning and development of the brain. Healthy skin, digestive system, organ and gland functions, the cardiovascular system and even the immune system all need these oils to work at their best. This is extremely important to body health.

Most everyone is oil deficient.

These oils are supplied to the diet with live raw organic foods, even when there are degenerative diseases taking place in the body, and one or more of these oils may be deficient in the body.

When recovering one's health, the key components in healing oils are flax seed oil or a combination of flax, sunflower, hemp and sesame oils, which are more commonly known as omega-3 and omega-9 fatty acids. These oils also include omega-6 fatty acids.

A good sign of the body needing oil supplements is when the skin is dry. When it is dry and flaky, the body needs more oil. Up to several tablespoons a day may be taken until the skin becomes soft and smooth again.

Once good oils are opened, they should be kept cool between each use. This keeps them from going rancid.

All cells need oils for their membranes.

Oils that have openings in their cellular structure are known as unsaturated oils or fats. Various nutrients can be absorbed into their molecules to be transported to the cells. They naturally have space to combine with nutrients and are known as "unsaturated "oils.

There are natural unsaturated fats in all the raw fruits, vegetables, and nuts and seeds.

Those fats that have no natural openings in their cells are known as **saturated fats**. They are our solid fats, at room temperature: meats, dairy, and eggs, etc. The body cannot use these fats and they become sticky and tend to stay in the arteries and linings of the body. They will eventually cause heart problems in the body when eaten often.

The fats that are **hydrogenated fats** are the ones that are really unsaturated fats, but have been hydrogenated to change he openings in their cell structure to make them solid at room temperatures. This process has heated the oils to a high temperature, destroying all the nutrients that were in the original oils, and making them useless to the body.

Some of these fats are lard, margarine, cooking oils, cheeses and of course peanut butter. They then become saturated fats, which means they have no openings in their cell structures to accept any nutrients. These oils have also been treated with such things as Drano, acids and bleach.

This long shelf life may be good for business, but very bad for body health. These products should not be consumed by anyone.

These trans-fatty acids are a huge contributor to heart and other diseases in the body.

Oils and butter should never be used for cooking, as they become very rancid once heated.

Their chemical structures are changed and they can not be used by the body.

Of course, if using strictly raw food in your diet, even butter as a dairy product is unacceptable.

Dairy products are also genetically modified and is possibly harmful to the body in the long term.

Another way to get your body good oils is by giving it raw nuts and seeds. They are high in oils and protein.

"Essential fatty acids and unsaturated fats are the good guys. Saturated fats or trans-fatty acids and hydrogenated oils are the bad guys," states Ron Garner in his book "*After the Doctors…What Can You Do?*"

What Are Supplements

Supplements are being taken by multitudes of people to make sure they are getting all the nutrients they need for their bodies, because our prepared foods are letting them down.

These supplements are lacking all the main nutrients that the body needs to function properly. This may be causing deficiencies in the body.

These supplements cannot be used by the body as they are mostly synthetic and composed of fillers.

They are dead to the body. This means they just get flushed through the body as expensive urination. They cannot replace any of the deficiencies that may be prevalent in the body, therefore people are still deficient in the nutrients the body needs.

The supplement industry has become a major player in freeing people from their money. The industry has not only bombarded us with media coverage on what is good for us, but has turned our doctors and practitioners into salesmen for them.

When you are lacking something in your body and you go buy these supplements, how do you know you are getting the correct vitamins or nutrients for your body?

Are they toxic to your body? Are they treating the right ailment? How do you know you are deficient of certain vitamins or minerals? The people selling these products are there to sell you products, not analyze your body to tell you what you are deficient in, or if that particular product can be used by your body.

It is live enzymes that heal, rebuild and revitalize your body, not synthetic supplements.

The body has to work very hard in order to get those supplements through your system. They are also very stimulating to the body and cause all kind of imbalances. This causes the body to use up important nutrients to rid itself of these dead supplements.

"All supplements are not created equal!! You simply must know what you are taking," says Ron Garner in his book
"*After the Doctors…What Can You Do?*"

The body can only work with one or two supplements at a time. Taking mega doses of supplements is usually not the answer. In fact you probably will still continue to get sicker.

If a person is living the raw food lifestyle, it will be that supplements are a thing of the past. The raw live foods will be healing the body for you in a totally natural way. You will not need any supplements to help you be well.

How wonderful that is. Saves you time, money and gives you better health.

Synthetic supplements are not used by the body therefore you are flushing them, without using them.

Natural supplements, such as raw food, are totally used by the body as FOOD!

Freshly Squeezed Juices

Juicing is one way to make your transition to raw food a pleasure. Juices are much easier for the body to assimilate and still give you all the nutrients that are needed by the body. They are absorbed into the blood stream immediately without having to be digested. They work quicker on the body and the body responds quicker.

Freshly squeezed fruit or vegetable juices are the best thing you can do for your health and well-being.

Fresh juices are living matter that has not been processed, denatured, heated or refined, and contain no additives.

Our body is a living organism and needs the nutrition that is natural and not in any way denatured. Unfortunately, this is the case with most foodstuffs available in supermarkets these days.

Drinking fresh juices will contribute markedly to your good health. It is never too late to change eating habits and to start a new healthy lifestyle.

Make drinking juices a regular habit and after a short while, you will experience the positive influence of these juices on your looks and vitality.

Juices bought in supermarkets often contain preservatives and other additives that should be avoided for health reasons. They are also highly processed.

Fresh juices purify your body, hydrate the body tissues, and supply you with vital nutrients and roughage, signaling repletion to the pituitary gland.

This indicates that you are satisfied and eat less, because the hunger is gone. This is one reason why the fresh juices are an ideal support to change eating habits and the first step towards a healthy, efficient, and slim body. Juices are easy to prepare and the combinations are endless for the optimum benefits.

You'll have to experiment to find the flavour combinations you like best. To get the freshest flavours while preserving the most nutrients, here are some tips.

Scrub It. While not all fruit and vegetables require peeling, many do. For example, the skins of oranges and grapefruits contain chemicals that can be toxic if consumed in large quantities. Waxed produce should be peeled before juicing, as should tropical fruits, which are often grown in countries where the use of pesticides isn't well regulated. Also, if you must buy non-organic fruits, be sure to wash them in a vinegar water bath before using.

Remove The Pits and Seeds. Apple seeds, which contain trace amounts of cyanide, should be removed before juicing. The seeds in melons, lemons, and limes and the pits from peaches, plums, and other stone fruits should also be removed. Grape seeds are safe, however, and can be placed in the juicer along with the fruit.

Use The Whole Vegetable. Most vegetables can be juiced in their entirety—leaves, stems, and all. Two exceptions are rhubarb and carrots. Rhubarb leaves and carrot tops both contain toxic compounds.

Chunk It. The openings of most juicers are quite small, so you should cut your produce into manageable pieces. Also small chunks put less strain on the motor, which will help your juicer last longer.

Blend Your Bananas. When juicing fruits or vegetables that contain little water, like bananas and avocados, it's helpful to juice other items first, then add the drier produce to produce a thick, smooth drink.

Sip It Quickly. Once the fruit or vegetable goes through the juicer, natural enzymes in the food begin to break down the nutrients. Juice loses nutritional value quickly. Moreover, its flavour is fleeting. For optimal benefits, drink juices within 30 minutes of making them.

Focus On Vegetables. While a tall glass of fruit juice can be a sweet treat, it is better to concentrate on vegetable juices. Fruit juices are too sugary and too *acidic to drink in large quantities. Vegetable juices are better nutritionally, and they have a higher *alkaline content.

Enjoy A Variety. For maximum healing benefits, drink juices from a variety of vegetables. The more variety you can work into your diet, the better. This is easy with juices, because you can combine several vegetables.

There are several manufacturers of **juicers on the market to make your juicing experience a joy.

When you experience several days receiving most of your nutrition from juices, not only do you get a higher portion of vitamins, minerals, and natural enzymes. Your body also doesn't have to work very hard at digestion, so you have more nutritionally rich blood with more time to clean up, heal overworked cells, and help the body to rejuvenate. You can also see an enhancement of your immune system. Excerpt from, *"Make your Juice Your Drugstore"* by Dr. L. Newman.
*See: Appendix C. **See: Appendix E *r*

About Sprouting

It is said that sprouts are the foods richest of nutrients. When the sprouts are shooting, it is the time of their highest energy and most complete nutrients. Live Enzymes abound in these sprouts.

Therefore, to become a sprouter in your new raw food lifestyle is a very good idea. Sprouts offer a tremendous amount of life force and a powerhouse of nutrition. Sprouts are vital and alive, as you will be when you eat them regularly. Adding sprouts to your diet is an easy way to gain energy, vitality, and good health.

Why eat sprouts? For many reasons:

• Healthy, economical and convenient
• Packed with nutrition
• Fresh, vital and alive all year round
• Inexpensive, fresh vegetables
• Easy to grow at home by anyone

Sprouts are living food. When seeds sprout, a tremendous amount of life force is released, and a powerhouse of nutrients are available to you.

Sprouts are an excellent source of enzymes, which are the "sparks of life" and help fight degenerative diseases. Seeds are packed with enough vitamins and minerals to initiate sprouting even before he roots pick up nutrients from the soil, and the leaves photosynthesize sunlight into energy. These nutrients are the freshest you can get, staying fresh until you start eating them. Sprouts do not need soil to grow.

Sprouts are most healthful when grown from certified organically raised seeds.

What do you need to begin sprouting?
Here's a list of supplies you will require:

• Organic sprouting seeds
• Measuring spoons
• Large wide mouthed jars with cheese-cloth/sprouter/or sprouting bags
• Cool, dry clean place to let them sprout in—usually a cupboard when it isn't too cool

Simple sprouting method:

1. Put seeds in large container and cover with about 3—4 times more water than seeds, to soak to increase mineral content—add piece of kelp or seaweed to your soak water (if you choose).

2. Soak according to *sprouting chart—usually from six to twelve hours.

3. After soaking, drain seeds well and put them in a **sprouting bag or large jar and spread them out and place the jar on its side at a 45 degree angle so the excess water can run off. Place the jar or sprouting bag in a cool, dark, clean place. If using a sprouting bag, put soaked seeds in bag and hang to drip with bowl under to catch the water. Rinse in clean water and squeeze out excess water and hang again. Do this twice daily—morning and evening.

4. Rinse and drain the sprouts three times daily using cool water. Generally in the morning, at noon, and in early evening. Always drain off excess water and shake the jar so the seeds are spread out and place the jar back on its side.

5. Once the sprouts have appeared, expose them to indirect sunlight for one or two days or until the leaves begin to turn green. Direct sunlight is much too hot for the sprouts. It may cook them.

6. Place finished sprouts in a large bowl of cool water and stir them around to remove the hulls and wash them.

7. Drain the sprouts and put them in a glass jar for up to seven to ten days in the refrigerator.

I have found through my experience that wide mouthed jars work very well for sprouting. Half-gallon jars seem to be a perfect fit for most sprouts. You may have to adjust the size of jar only by the size of family you have. A *sprouting chart is included in this book for your use. For sprouting bags go to www.liverawkitchen.com

Apart from humans, domestic pets are the only animals that eat cooked food. Yes, it is right to feed your best friends the same raw food, sprouts, etc. that you yourself would eat. The animals in our lives, tend to suffer the same disease that humans do, therefore, the raw foods, seeds, sprouts, etc. will also help to clean up their diseases. This also makes up for the nutritional deficiencies in the pet foods on the market today, and your pet will probably thank you for it.

Getting
Into
It

You do not have to become a raw food eater, you already are one. Nature constructed us to utilize and replenish the body by eating alive, raw foods.

This you can prove by just watching your body changes, when you begin to use alive, raw foods again in your diet.

Your body will become alive, vital and energetic without you doing anything else. Your body will heal and rejuvenate all on its own. Give it that chance.

There is a basic guideline you may want to follow to assure your complete nutrition for each day. You should eat each day:

• Fresh fruits
• leafy green vegetables
• nuts and/or seeds

Always eat your fruits alone, preferably one kind at a time. This way your body will know when it gets enough.

You will learn to listen to your body and what it needs. I found when a food became distasteful to me, my body no longer needed the kind of nourishment it was giving me, and would not taste good. Therefore another nutrient was needed, and my body would crave or like a different food, for its nutrients.

You will want to eat your nuts and seeds with your leafy green veggies, because they assimilate into your body easier with the enzymes from your greens.

The protein from your nuts and seeds will be used better by your body. The nuts and seeds should be ground lightly, or chewed very well.

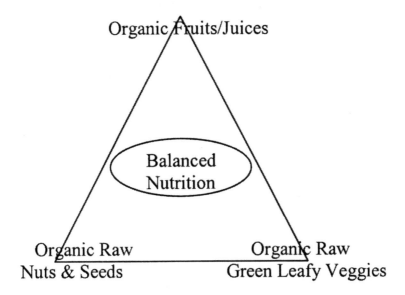

Raw Food Triangle

If these basic guidelines are followed each day, your body will get the nutrients it needs.

Your dressings should be made with oils, such as flaxseed oil, sesame seed oil, hemp oil, extra-virgin olive oil, or walnut oil. These will give you your required amounts of omega-3 fatty acids your body will require. A large percentage of the population has an imbalance of omega-3 and omega 6 fats in their bodies.

We are all overloaded with omega-6 fats from all the red meats and dairy products we are using today. This imbalance is making it very difficult for our bodies to use these fats. They are very difficult to break down as they become settled in our veins and organs to give us problems.

This is easily changed, by changing the fats we use on a daily basis.

Change your omega-6 fats for omega-3 fats and not only the bad fats will be moved out of your body, but the bad acids will also be removed. These are the primary reasons we have so much of the population with arthritis, bad joints, etc., These acidic fats settle in the joints and muscles and cause pain and deterioration in these areas later on in life.

We eat food to supply our bodies with nutrition. Real food for the body contains, and is broken down by the digestive process into the usable components of:

• Glucose—for energy
• Protein—for building and repairing tissue
• Fatty Acids—to construct membranes, and move electrical currents
• Minerals—are catalysts and building components
• Enzymes—(vitamins) are catalysts
• Water—the medium for chemical processes.

Dr. Robbins says: Raw foods for the body must be something:

1. Edible & grown by nature of the plant kingdom.

2. Plants, which can be eaten without processing in any way.

3. An entire meal of just that one substance can be eaten and thoroughly enjoyed.

Raw foods have everything in them that the body needs, to be healthy.

The body can assimilate these and use them to clean and rejuvenate the body.

Raw foods are alkaline, but once they are cooked they become acid foods toxic to the body. Cooking destroys the nutrients of the foods and the body can no longer use them. It considers them poison.

Processed foods, which our shelves are full of these days, are full of preservatives, chemicals and by-products that our bodies cannot assimilate, therefore they are difficult for the body to get rid of. Most of them are to enhance the flavour of our foods, so we will like them and go back for more. We become addicted to flavours.

When our body is not given the essential nutrients, the body must find them somewhere, and therefore is using up your "warehouse" of enzymes.

In other words it has to feed off itself in order to be able to digest, assimilate and rejuvenate, to do its job. The body has to work very hard in order to rid the body of these toxins from these processed foods, and it begins to deteriorate with time.

The body can only do one job at a time.

If the body is cleaning and rebuilding and a toxin or toxins are introduced to the body, it must abandon its present job to rid itself of the deadly toxins just introduced. It is more important to get them out of the system as quickly as possible.
These toxins are deadly to the body and they must be eliminated before the body can go back to its work of cleaning and rebuilding.

When you feel you have a surge of energy after drinking a coffee, the body makes an anti-caffeine agent in your body to combat the caffeine you are putting in your body. Therefore, this anti-caffeine agent is what gives you the surge. This action is very difficult on the body, as it takes a lot of energy and nutrition to do this. That is why your energy surge doesn't last very long, and you may become tired.

Watch the sulphur in your dried fruits. Sulphur in the body forces it to go below its normal functions and it is very dangerous.

Watch soy food it is a by-product and should not be eaten by anyone. They are the most genetically engineered products on the market today. All soy products are treated the same way. Soy is also acid to the system.

Be sure to check your labels before buying, to be sure there are no ingredients in the things you are buying, that you do not want to eat.

Now that you have started changing the way you are eating, you will be putting different foods together in different ways. **Don't be afraid to experiment.** Everyone has a different food appeal, so be brave and put the things together that appeal to you.

Using these five flavours in your recipes will make your food very tasty and nutritious. They are:

• Sour
• Sweet
• Salty
• Spicy
• Bitter

For the **sour taste** you would use: lemons, rhubarb, lemon grass, sorrel

For the **sweet taste** you would use: dried fruits such as figs, dates, raisins, prunes, fresh fruits such as banana, mango, peach, pears, apple juice, orange juice, or honey

For the **salty taste** you would use: Celtic Sea Salt, sea vegetables such as kelp, dulse, nori, arame, celery, parsley, dill, or cilantro.

For the **spicy taste** you would use: garlic leaves or cloves, onion leaves or bulbs, radish, horse radish, cayenne pepper, mustard greens or seeds, ginger, wasabe, sea weed, dry or fresh herbs such as basil, dill, cinnamon, nutmeg, cilantro, rosemary, or peppermint.

For a **bitter taste** you would use: poultry seasoning or cayenne pepper, dandelion, onion, garlic, bay leaf, sage, celery tops, endive or parsley.

Some other helpful hints to use in your preparations are as follows:

When recipes call for:

Nuts, Seeds and Grains: use almonds, walnuts, filberts, cashews, pine nuts, pecans, sunflower seeds, flaxseed, sesame seed,

Dried Fruits: use pitted prunes, raisins, apricots, dates, figs or currants.

Fresh fruits and Berries: use blueberries, apples, bananas, pineapple, mango, apricots, raspberries, cranberries, blackberries, peaches, or papayas.

The sky is the limit. If your body wants it, eat it. Your taste buds will become very enhanced. Raw food will taste wonderful.

For your start on the Raw Food lifestyle, included are some recipes for you to use. Have fun with them and use them only as a guideline if you choose, while making your own recipes up.

The life of the earth and sun is being given to you through these enriched live foods. Always learn from Nature.

The most important thing is to have fun with this. Enjoy your journey to renewed health. The choice is yours to make.

Be patient, persevere and be consistent, and you will become what you want to be. **I DID !!**

And remember I am always here for the support you may need or the questions you may have.

Substitutes
For
Cravings

Below are some of the substitutes you can use in place of cooked food cravings or junk food habits.

Craving French fries, mashed potatoes, or potato chips—replace with nuts and sea weed, use "Instead of Potatoes" Recipe.

Salt craving—replace with seaweed such as Wakame or Bull Kelp. By mixing these with almonds, you are getting a tasty protein treat, and the seaweed has all the minerals and trace minerals you require. Chopped up avocado with sea salt. Is also a great protein

Celery ground and dried is a good salt substitute.

Pastries, pies, cakes, candy and cookies—replace with raisins, dates, nuts and sunflower seeds, mixed together as treat, cookies from fruit juicer pulp. Grind nuts, or just add honey and sea salt to cup of nuts.

Use "Date Treat" recipe in the Recipe section: Must Miscellaneous.

Ice Creams, Cheesecakes, etc—replace with frozen fruit ice cream, and lemon puddings or lemon cream.

Milk/Milkshakes—replace with nut milks, and nut milk smoothies, cantaloupe milk smoothie.

Meats—replace with vegetable sushi, nut sushi, nut loafs, etc.

Chocolate—replace with raw carob chocolate cake, raw carob treats, "Date Treats"

Salad Dressings—replace with raw salad dressings, Lemon or Lime juice, or Oils

Cheese—replace with nut or seed cheese, tahini cheese(make your own)

Drugs & Alcohol—replace with sunflower seeds, green juice, "Date Treats."

Bread—replace with flax seed crackers, nutty treats

Recipes
My Favourites
Both Collected and
My Own Creations

All Made and Tested
In My Own Kitchen

These recipes are all easy and tasty and help you serve exciting and nutritious meals. They were made with the five flavours in mind. You will notice that each time you make up the same recipe, you may end up with a different taste or texture. This is because the raw organic fruits or vegetables you are using may be different from the last time you used them.

They may be riper, greener, grown differently, etc. This all affects the texture and flavour of the foods. This makes each dish a new experience, even though you have made it before with the same recipe.

Quick Tips

Dry Soup Mix

Chop to size required and dry until dried
to store. Store in freezer.
Parsley
Onion
Carrots
Celery
When using, add handful to bowl of
WARM water & let sit for a few minutes to
soften.

Add:
1 tsp. Olive Oil
1/4 tsp. Sea Salt to taste

Sea Weed For Salads
Dill Weed
Dulse or Nori
Dried Ground Ginger
Flax Seed, ground

Trail Mix

Dried Fruit
Nuts
Coconut, fresh
Dates, Raisins, etc

Popcorn

Small Seeds, like:
Sunflower Seeds
Sesame Seeds
Soak for 4 hours Dehydrate until dry.
Substitute for popcorn

Nut Snack

Take your favourite pitted Dates.
Push Almonds or other nuts into the pit
holes. Eat. Tasty & nutritious.

Salt

Dehydrate chopped celery until dry.
Blend to powder. 20 lbs. of celery=1 quart
of powder for salt.

Sugar

Dehydrate finely chopped Jicama until
dried. Blend to powder for sugar.

Quickie Dressing

Equal amounts of:
Honey
Olive Oil
Lemon Juice
Shake to mix well before serving.

Tasty
Yummy
Milks,
Cheeses,
Creams
And
Yogurts

Almond Milk/Cream or Yogurt

makes 1 litre
1 cup whole Almonds, (soaked in 3 cups of water for 12 hours) drained & rinsed 2-3 cups pure Water

After soaked almonds are strained, pour boiling water over them and let sit for exactly 30-seconds—NO LONGER. Pour off and remove skins. Gives you a nice white product.

Put almonds in blender with 2-3 cups of water and puree until smooth & creamy.

Pour puree through a fine mesh bag or milk bag to remove pulp.

After pressing out all the milk from the pulp, use the pulp in other recipes like Ricotta Cheese, Zesty Cheese or Choice Cheesecake.

For cream, or yogurt, add 1-2 cups of water to the soaked almonds, or enough for the consistency you want, blend until smooth.

You can make yogurt with the milk by leaving it sit out on the counter for 4-5 days to ferment. Less time if the weather is warm.

Make yogurt before adding sweetener. To make whipped cream, use less water with nuts, puree until creamy smooth

Zesty Almond Cheese

Pulp from Almond milk
1/2 cup Olive Oil
1/4 cup Lemon juice
1/2 tsp. Sea Salt
1/2 cup Dill Weed or Green
Onions, chopped

Mix all together & let sit for a few hours to ferment and meld the flavours some. Should be fairly firm.

Great on crackers.

Almond Ricotta Cheese

3/4 cup firm Almond pulp
1/4 cup red Onion, minced
1/2 small clove Garlic, crushed
dash of Nutmeg
1/2 tsp. Sea Salt or to taste

Combine ingredients, adding water if needed to achieve desired consistency.

Can be stored in fridge, up to 1 week.

Serve as a spread or a dip.

Fetty Almond Cheese

3/4 cup very firm Almond pulp
1/2 small clove Garlic, crushed
1/2 tsp. Lemon juice
1/2 tsp. Sea Salt
dash of Nutmeg
dash of White Pepper

Combine ingredients for cheese and mix well. Spoon into a cheese cloth lined colander & place weight on top.
(A plastic bag filled with beans work well.)

Allow to remain in fridge another 12 hours.

Use in salads & other feta cheese recipes.

Almond Whipped Cream

1 cup soaked, skinned Almonds
1/2-1 cup purified Water

Be careful to use only enough water to keep the blender moving, to make a smooth cream

Add:
1/2-1 Banana
1 tsp. Vanilla Bean

Serve with fruit & pies.

Make Sour Cream by replacing the Cane Sugar and Vanilla Bean with 1 Tbsp. Lemon Juice, or more to taste, or Lime juice

Mock Sour Cream

1 cup Sunflower Seeds
(soaked 8-12 Hours)
1 tsp. minced Garlic
1 tsp. Sea Salt
1/2 cup chopped Cucumber
(peeled & seeded)
1 Tbsp. or more Water
1/4 cup Celery juice
1/2 Lemon (peeled, seeded &
chopped)
1/4 cup chopped Onion

In a blender, combine the cucumber with the celery juice & liquefy. Add the sunflower seeds and blend until smooth.

Add the onion, lemon, garlic & sea salt; blend until smooth, adding enough water to achieve the desired consistency.

Refrigerate until needed or, for more authentic sour cream taste, cover with cheese cloth & leave container on counter until slightly fermented. Depending on the temperature, this may take 4-8 hours Yields 1 1/2 cups.

Nut and /or Seed Milks
Cheeses/Yogurts

2 cups of any nuts or seeds combined
3-4 cups water

Soak the nuts and seeds in water over night. In morning, drain off water and put seeds in blender. Add enough water to double the amount of seeds.

Blend until smooth and put in a milk bag and hang or squeeze until all the moisture or liquid has been taken off. Use as the milk or let sit for yogurt.

Transfer the pulp to a bowl and either let ferment for a while, or make into your favorite cheese right away.

For Yogurt: Let the milk ferment, sitting on the cupboard, at room temperature for at least 8-12 hours Add your favorite fruit if you like, and enjoy. Will ferment faster in warm weather.

For Milk Bags go to LiveRawKitchen.com/index.php

Here are some suggestions for nut & seed combinations:

• Almonds & Sesame
• Pecans & Almonds
• Pecans & Sesame
• Sesame & Hazelnuts
• Sunflower & Almond
• Walnuts & Pine Nuts

These combinations really make a nice yogurt as well as milks. Follow instructions above.

Use the pulp from the above combinations to make your cheese. You can also make a Cheesecake from the pulps.
Recipe on page 242.

Joyful
Juices

Here are some juice combinations you may like to try, or experiment and put together your own combinations.

Smoothie Orange Drink

2 Tbsp. Flax seeds, soaked 1-2 hours in
1/4 cup Water
8-10 Oranges, peeled
2 Romaine lettuce leaves

Soak flax seeds & chill in refrigerator.
Juice the peeled oranges. Save some for garnishing.

In blender, puree 1 cup of orange juice with the flax seed and romaine until smooth.

Then blend in remaining juice.

Serve in fancy glasses if you like and garnish with orange wedges.

Fresh Apple Juice

3 large Apples, washed and cored.

Fresh Tropical Blend

1 Guava, peeled and pitted
1 Papaya
1 Pineapple slice, skinned
1 large Orange, peeled, pitted
1 Mango, peeled, pitted

Blend & enjoy!

Cantaloupe Milk Smoothie

Take cantaloupe, cut into chunks, put in a blender, add enough water to cover cantaloupe. Then blend on high until whipped up and has smooth creamy consistency.

Fresh Carrot Juice

5 large Carrots washed, topped and tailed. Leave skin on for more vitamins & minerals

Energy Boost

1 Carrot washed, topped and tailed
1 Celery stalk with leaves, washed
1 Beet root, skin washed, leave on roots & tops
Parsley, a few loose leaves washed & rolled
Lettuce, a few loose leaves, washed & rolled
Watercress, a few loose leaves, washed & rolled
Spinach, a few loose leaves, washed & rolled

3 Tomatoes, washed and stemmed
Salt to taste
Blend all and en

Fresh Melon Combo

Try a combination of 3 different types of Melon:
Cantaloupe
Watermelon
Honeydew

Remove skins and seeds and cut into manageable pieces that will fit into the juicer chute.

Fresh Celery Juice

1 head of Celery
1 large Carrot washed, topped and tailed a small wedge of Lemon peeled and seeded

Fresh Cucumber and Carrot Juice

2 large Carrots, washed, topped and tailed
1 medium Cucumber, washed
Blend and Enjoy!

Fresh Carrot, Apple and Ginger Juice

2 medium Carrots, washed, unpeeled,
topped and tailed
1 crisp Apple, washed, seeded and quartered
1 inch of fresh root Ginger, peeled

The more ginger you add the spicier it gets!

Fresh Pineapple and Carrot Juice

4 large Carrots, washed, topped and tailed
1/4 of a Pineapple, skin removed
Blend and Enjoy.

Grapefruit, Ginger, Apple Juice

1 Grapefruit, peeled, leaving most of the white pulp intact.
1/2 inch of Ginger, not peeled
3 golden delicious Apples, cored
(these help counteract the tartness of the grapefruit)

Apple, Blueberry Juice

1 cup fresh Blueberries (or frozen) funneled into juicer alternating
with 4 Apples (so blueberries do not escape)

Carrot, Spinach, Apple, Beet Juice

8 Carrots
handful of Spinach
3 Apples
1/4 of Beet without greens
Juice and Enjoy.

Carrot, Parsley, Spinach, Celery, Apple Juice

8 Carrots
handful of Parsley
handful of Spinach
2 Apples
2 stalks of Celery

Put in juicer. Alternate carrots and apples with greens to keep them moving through juicer.

Green Lemonade

1 granny smith Apple (or green apple)
1/2 of large Lemon, peel too
3/4 inch fresh Ginger

Blend and pour over ice. Also makes a great frozen treat. Delightful.

Energy Boost

6 Carrots
handful of Parsley

Holiday Treat

1 slice Lemon peel
1 large bunch of Grapes
2 Apples

Bedtime Snack

1 Pear
2 Apples

Cleanser

1 Beet
1/2 Cucumber
4 Carrots

Boost Your Alkaline

3 stalks of Celery
1/4 head Cabbage (red or green)

Memory Sparkler

1/4 Lemon (peel if not organic) optional
1/4 head of small Cabbage, cut to fit juicer
3 stalks of Celery with leaves
4-5 medium sized Carrots

Wash and top the carrots scrub well
Wash celery & cabbage
Juice all, add lemon if desired, stir & pour.

Liver Tonic

1/2 Beet
2-3 Carrots

For Potassium

1 handful of Spinach
1 handful of Parsley
2 stalks of Celery
4-6 Carrots

Power Zap

Drink this about 15 minutes before your meal.

1 tart organic Apple, washed, unpeeled, quartered copped
3-5 organic Carrots, scrubbed, unpeeled
2 stalks of organic Kale, cleaned, stems removed
Juice & drink.

Eye Opener

1/2 Fennel
2 stalks Celery
1/2 Cucumber
1 large Apple, organic, unpeeled
handful of Spinach
handful of Parsley
juice of 1/2 Grapefruit

Great for removing the cobwebs in the morning.

Fruit Cocktail

Juice together:

2 Nectarines or Peaches
1/2 Cantaloupe
2 Apples
1 inch Ginger root
2 Tbsp. Ground Flax seed
Add 8-10 ozs. of ice cubes and mix.

Serve in fancy wine glass, with sliver of ginger on rim

Lunch Break

1 Beet
2 Cucumbers
2 stalks Celery
4 Carrots

Digestion Helper

1/4 Lemon with peel
1/2 Grapefruit peeled
2 Oranges

Green Drink Life's Life Blood

Use any of the following ingredients:

Dark leafy greens (Romaine, Chard, Kale,
Parsley, Cilantro, etc)
Cucumber
Celery
Carrots (if it's hard to get down without a sweetener, we use pure
Carrot juice or Carrot/Apple juice as a chaser)
Onion and/ or Garlic for flavour
Ginger for flavour
Lemon or lime for flavour

Mix & drink.
Increases the health of your cells.

Another Green Drink

Combine:

4 oz. Buckwheat sprout juice
4 oz. Sunflower sprout juice
4 oz. Alfalfa sprout juice
1 Carrot juiced
1 Scallion juiced
2 Tbsp. Sauerkraut juice

You can combine this drink with your juice fasting and have it 2 times daily, morning and evening, along with plenty of fruit and vegetable juices, and at least 16 ozs. of water every two hours.

This should be done each Sunday or once weekly, as it suits your time schedule.

There are other Green Drinks you can use as well, that are full of enzymes and nutrients.

Enzyme and Chlorophyl Booster

Take at least 6 leaves of, or combination of the following leafy greens:

Kale
Romaine
Bok Choy
Spinach
Swiss Chard
Red Leaf Lettuce, etc

Roll these leaves up into a tight roll and put through your juicer.

You should get about 1/4 cup of juice.

Add 1/4 cup of water to juice.
Drink 1/2 cup of this juice in morning hours and 1/2 cup of this juice in afternoon, before dinner hour
Do not keep juice for the day.
Remake more juice for afternoon drink.

Breakfast Beckons

Besides having the juices mentioned in the last chapter, most breakfasts are fresh fruits. One may also add the following breakfasts to your menu.

Breaky Goodie

Toss:

1/2 cup of Grapes, washed
1/2 cup Strawberries, washed, de-stemmed
1/2 cup Kiwi fruit, halved

With:
1 Tbsp. Lime juice
1 Tbsp. Honey

Sunny Muesli

1 cup organic, whole Buckwheat kernels
3/4 cup Almond or Nut milk
1/4 cup Raisins

Put buckwheats and raisins in bowl and cover with nut milk. Cover bowl with cloth and let sit overnight.

In morning stir, and add:
1 Tbsp. Honey
1 Tbsp. Lemon juice (optional)
1 Tbsp. Nuts, ground or grated (optional.)

Fresh fruit may also be sliced and added to serving.

Melon Morning

Take:
Watermelon
Muskmelon
Cantaloupe
Honeydew Melon

Make into balls and combine in bowl.
Add:
1 Tbsp. Honey
1 Tbsp. Lime Juice

Combine and pour into bowl with melons and mix until covered. You may also sprinkle with a bit of dried, shredded coconut. Enjoy.

Boastful
Breads,
Buns
and
Crackers

Flaxseed Crackers, Buns or Bread

Grind 2 cups of Flaxseed in a grinder and set aside.

Blend:
1 cup Water
1 large Onion, chopped
3 stalks of Celery, chopped
4 cloves of Garlic, medium
1 tsp. Caraway seed
1 tsp. Coriander seed
1 tsp. Sea Salt

Mix ground flaxseed into blended mix by hand. Mix thoroughly. Cover the dough with a cloth and let sit overnight on the counter to ferment slightly.

Using a spatula, spread thinly on non-stick sheet in dehydrator and divide into desired size squares. Dehydrate until dry and crispy.
Will keep for a couple of months.

Makes about 30 crackers.
Enjoy

Cool Flax Crackers/ Buns or Bread

1 cup ground Flaxseed
1 cup Walnuts, soaked overnight
1 cup chopped Celery
2 tsps. Caraway seed, soaked overnight
2 Tbsps. Coriander seed
1 medium to large Onion
1/2 cup Water
1/2 cup Olive Oil
1/2 cup Raisins
1/2 Lemon, juiced
1 tsp. Sea Salt

Blend the Walnuts & Onion in food processor until finely chopped.

Put in bowl and mix in Flaxseed by hand.

Blend Celery, Olive Oil, Raisins, Water in blender.

Combine both mixtures.

Add Sea Salt, Coriander, Lemon Juice, Caraway and mix thoroughly.

Shape into desired buns or loaves, or spread thinly for crackers, and dry for required time in dehydrator. You want to flip the loaves or buns, about every 3-4 hours to dry evenly on both sides

Enjoy.

Sprouted Grain Crisps

2 cups mixed Buckwheat Sprouts (*soaked overnight and sprouted for 1 day)
1 Tbsp. Onion, chopped
1/2 tsp. Garlic crushed garlic clove
1 tsp. Sea Salt to taste
Water, to keep food processor mixing
Sesame or Poppy Seeds to roll crackers in.

Combine ingredients, except seeds, in food processor. Chop until well mixed.

Form into buns or loaves, or spread on dehydrator sheets for crackers, and sprinkle with seeds.

Allow to dehydrate for 12-24 hours Turn buns or loaves every 3-4 hours to dry evenly.

Store covered, in a cool, dark place.

*See sprouting direction on page

Sprouted Crackers

1/2 cup each of Buckwheat & Sunflower seeds
(*Soak over night, sprout for 24-36 hours)
Ground slightly, to break kernels, put aside

Mix:
2 tsp. Caraway seed
2 tsp. Coriander seed
1 cup Celery, chopped
1 large Onion
2 tsp. Sea Salt

4 cloves of Garlic, mashed

Put in food processor and mix until smooth. Add ground grains by hand & mix well. Let sit overnight to ferment a little.

Spread on dehydrator sheets and score before drying.

Dry for about 8-12 hours. Or until the crispness you like.

Buckwheat Sticks

1/2 cup of Buckwheat ground
1/4 cup Flaxseed, ground
1/4 cup Caraway seeds
1/2 cup Sunflower seeds
1/2 cup Raisins
1/2 cup Celery, chopped
1 Onion
3 cloves Garlic

Soak above seeds overnight to soften.
Rinse in morning and process in food processor, with raisins, celery, onion, garlic.

Add some water if you want to make crackers to make the batter thinner to spread

Add in 1 Tbsp. Indian Spice Mix, or more to taste.

Roll out into 6-7 inch bread sticks. and put into dehydrator and dry for 6-8 hours depending on the crispness you want.

Sassy Soups

Tasty Thai Soup

11/2 cups chopped Cucumbers
3/4 cup Olive Oil
3 cups Water
1/2 cup Lemon juice
1 cup Dates or Raisins
1/2 tsp Turmeric
1/2 Spicy Pepper
11/2 Red Pepper
1 cup fresh Basil or Parsley

Blend until smooth & creamy.
Adjust flavour to your liking.

This soup can be made with Kohlrabi in place of the cucumber.

Garden Green Soup

1 Avocado
1 cup Water
2 unwaxed Cucumbers
1 cup Spinach
2 Green Onions
1 clove Garlic

1/3 Yellow Bell Pepper
Kelp to taste
Fresh Mint Leaves

In blender, puree 1/2 of the water & the avocado. Then add rest of ingredients, except mint & kelp.

Blend to desired thickness & thinning with the remaining water.

Flavour with dulse or kelp to taste.
Serve and garnish with mint leaves

Spicey Soup

3/4 cups Celery & leaves,
chopped
21/2 cups Water
1/2 tsp. Sea Salt
1/8 cup Olive Oil
1/4 cup Lemon juice
1/4 cup Raisins (Honey, Dates
also are good)
Spicy Pepper to taste
1/2 cup Basil, or bunch
1/2 Red Pepper chopped
handful diced Carrots

Put all ingredients in blender & mix until smooth.
Serves 4.

Carrot Beet Soup

3/4 cup chopped Carrots
1/2 cup Olive Oil
21/2 cups water

1/2 tsp. Sea Salt
1/4 Spicy Pepper
1/2 cup Lemon juice
1/2 cup Raisins
1/2 cup Basil or Parsley diced
handful, diced Beets
handful Red Pepper, sliced

Put all in blender & blend until smooth.
Serve with crackers of your choice.

Green Goddess Soup

2-3 stalks Celery
1 Avocado
1 Red Pepper
3-4 cups Broccoli
1/2 Onion
2-3 cups Water
Kelp, Sea Salt or Dulse to taste
1/2 cup Parsley

In a blender, puree the celery, avocado, onion, pepper, broccoli & parsley until very smooth. (Add more water if you want a thinner soup.)

Add Sea Salt, Dulse or kelp to taste.

This would also be good with the Indian Spice Mix as seasoning.

Garnish with a lemon circle floating on top and serve.

Calcium Soup

20 Pumpkin Seeds
3 Tbsp. flax Oil
1/2 tsp. Sea Salt
2 Yellow Peppers
1 Red Pepper
1 Avocado
2 Lemons
1/3 of Red Onion
2 cloves Garlic
1 handful Parsley
10 kale Leaves
(dinosaur kale, preferably)

Peel the lemons, leaving the white pulp intact. Blend all ingredients, adding water as you blend to make a smooth, rich, thick consistency.

Selective
Salads

Salad Greens

You can pretty well use anything for salad greens but iceberg lettuce, which really doesn't have any nutrient value. All should be bought "Organic." Some of the more popular are:

Arugula
Beet Greens
Bok Choy
Celery
Chinese Greens of all kinds
Cilantro
Dandelion Greens
Mustard Greens
Parsley
Red Leaf Lettuce
Romaine Lettuce
Spinach
Turnip Greens

To name just as few.
Enjoy.

It is suggested to include your nuts and seeds with your salad greens. Adding them to your salads gives variety and texture to your salads. It is preferred to grind them first. They also will be assimilated and digested easier if eaten this way.

You can also add different fruits to your salad greens for a different flavour and texture. Don't be afraid to experiment.

Dreamy Wild Salad

4-5 Handfuls of Wild Greens;
like Dandelion, Mustard, Lambs
Quarters, etc
2 Avocados
40 Olives
4 tsp. Extra-Virgin Olive Oil

Mix the Greens, Olives together
with 1 Avocado, diced. Mash other
Avocado and add Olive Oil to it,
mixing well.

Pour over Salad Greens.

You may also put all Avocado in salad & dribble Oil over for dressing.

Sweet and Tart Salad

3 cups shredded Cabbage
11/2 cups chopped Apple
1/2 cup or to taste Celery Seed Dressing

Shred cabbage very thinly and toss together cabbage & apple. Pour on dressing and toss lightly to coat evenly. Dressing below goes very well with this salad.

Celery Seed Dressing

1/4 cup Honey
1 tsp. Dry Mustard
1 tsp. sea salt
41/2 Tbsp. Lemon Juice
1 tsp. grated Onion
1 cup Flax seed Oil
1 Tbsp. Celery seed

Mix honey, mustard and salt. Blend in 2 tablespoons of the Lemon Juice, and the grated onion. Gradually beat in the flax seed oil. Beat until thick & slowly beat in the remaining Lemon Juice. Stir in celery seed.
Pour into screw top jar. Cover tightly and shake vigorously to blend well.
Store covered in refrigerator.
Shake well before using.

Dressing/ Marinade

3/4 cup Flaxseed oil
1/2 tsp. Celtic Sea Salt
2 Tbsp. Liquid Honey
1 tsp. Organic Basil
1 tsp. Organic Thyme
1 tsp. Organic Oregano
1/2 tsp. Cayenne Pepper
1/4 cup Lemon juice

Whisk all dressing ingredients together in a jar with a lid.

Pour 1/2 of the marinade over the bean salad and let marinade in fridge overnight. Save rest of dressing for other use.
Dressing may also be used over

Baby Green Salad Mixture.

As with all dressings, store covered in refrigerator and shake well before using.

Red Pepper Cucumber Salad

Dressing:
1/4 cup Almond cream
1/4 cup Mock Sour Cream
1 Tbsp. Lime juice

Salad:
2 Red Peppers thinly sliced
1 small English Cucumber, seeded,
thinly sliced
3 Tbsp. Finely chopped Scallions
3 Tbsp. Fresh Dill

Whisk dressing ingredients in large bowl until blended.

Add remaining ingredients, stir gently to mix and coat.

Serve.

Pepper & Cauliflower Salad

1 Yellow Pepper, thinly sliced in strips
1 Red Pepper, thinly sliced in strips
1/2 head of Cauliflower, cut into florets
2 Tbsp. Extra Virgin Olive Oil
Sea Salt to taste
Black Olives
Almond Feta Cheese
2 Tbsp. fresh Parsley, chopped

Dressing:
1/4 cup Extra Virgin Olive Oil
1 Tbsp. Lemon juice (fresh)
2 Garlic cloves, chopped
2 tsp. Fennel seeds
Sea salt to taste
White Pepper to taste

Base:
4 cups mixed Baby greens

Place pepper & cauliflower in bowl
Mix with olive oil & salt.
Mix dressing and add to vegetables.

Put on greens on serving plate and sprinkle with chopped parsley, add olives, and almond cheese. Serve at once.

Greek Salad

Dressing:
1 Tbsp. Flax Oil or Extra Virgin
Olive Oil
2 Tbsp. Water

1 Tbsp. Lemon juice
1 tsp. whole dried Oregano
1/2 tsp. Sea Salt, or to taste

Combine ingredients for dressing and set aside.

Salad:
4 medium Red Peppers, cut into large chunks
1 Cucumber, cut in half lengthwise, seeded and sliced crosswise
1 large Yellow Pepper, cut into quarters and sliced
1 small Red Onion, sliced thin
1/2 head Romaine Lettuce, washed and broken into pieces
24 Black Olives
1/2 cup Almond Feta Cheese, cut into
1/2 inch cubes

Combine ingredients, except cheese, and add dressing and toss well. Serve on individual plates and add cheese.
Serve immediately.

Zesty Coleslaw

4 cups shredded Cabbage
4 carrots, grated
2 sweet Red Peppers, thinly sliced
2 Oranges, peeled, quartered, seeded
1 medium Red Onion, sliced thinly
1/2 cup chopped Parsley
1/4 cup chopped fresh Basil
1 Tbsp. Orange zest
2 Tbsp. slivered Almonds

In large bowl combine all ingredients, except almonds. Toss well.
Add Avo-Mayonaise (recipe following).
Toss again. Sprinkle with almond slivers.

Avo Mayonaise

1 Avocado
1-2 Garlic cloves
1/2 tsp. Sea Salt
1/4 cup Lemon juice
1/2 tsp. white or Red Pepper

Cut avocado in pieces and put in blender with lemon juice. Blend until smooth.
Add rest of ingredients and blend until smooth again. Put into salad or use as dip.

Easy Thai Salad

4 Cucumbers, peeled, cut in thin circles
juice of 1 Lemon
1 bunch Dill
1 bunch Cilantro
1 med. Onion
3 tsp. Curry powder
1 tsp. Sea Salt or to taste
3 Tbsp. Honey
1/3 cup Olive oil
1 cup Sunflower seeds (soaked for 2 hrs)

Peel & slice the cucumbers into thin circles and transfer to bowl. Finely chop the cilantro & dill and mix with the cucumbers. Add the onion, lemon juice & olive oil.
Finish by adding the rest of the ingredients & mixing well.

Silicon Salad

1 head Romaine lettuce
4 Cucumbers
6 Okra
2 Red Bell Peppers
3 Tbsp. Horsetail herb
1 Avocado or 1 ounce of
Extra Virgin Olive Oil

Cut, dice, mix in a salad. Add Avocado or Olive Oil for dressing.

Great salad to relieve brittle fingernails, keeps hair from turning grey, the pain of tendonitis, ligament and tendon inflammation.

Delicious Dressings

Almond Mayonnaise

Make this mayonnaise, using your Almond
Sour Cream recipe.

Using 1 cup of Almond Sour Cream, add:

2-3 Tbsp. Lemon juice, or to taste
1 tsp. of herbs, such as:
Basil, Indian Spice Mix, Oregano,
Cayenne,
Parsley, or Onion
1 Tbsp. Honey or to taste

Mix all the ingredients well and pour over coleslaw salad.

Dilly Dressing

1 Cucumber
1/4 cup Olive Oil
1/2 cup Lemon Juice
1/2 cup Dill Weed
2 stalks Celery
1 tsp. Organic Mustard powder (Fresh Mustard Seed Ground)

Process all the ingredients in a blender until creamy. Thin with water if you would like a thinner dressing. Serve on your favourite Salad.

Vegetable Marinade

1 tsp. Sea Salt
6 Tbsp. Lemon juice
4 Tbsp. Olive Oil

1 Tbsp. Honey
2 cloves Garlic
1 tsp. Dry Mustard (Fresh Organic Mustard Seed Ground)
1 tsp. Paprika
1 tsp. White Pepper

Sliced Onion
Red Pepper julienned
Sliced Carrot

Place all ingredients in bowl and mix well. Add to vegetables and coat well.

Cover and put in fridge for at least 2 hours or overnight before serving, to let the flavours meld.

Also very good with zucchini slices julienne style.

Blueberry Salad Dressing

1/2 cup Blueberries (fresh or frozen)
1/4 cup Flax Seed Oil
1/3 cup Lemon Juice
dash of Celtic Sea Salt
1 Tbsp. Unpasteurized Honey

Blend ingredients with a hand mixer or whisk. If whisking, mash the blueberries first. Pour over mixed baby greens and enjoy.

Easy Avocado Dressing

In blender mix one Avocado with the fresh squeezed juice of Orange.

Pour onto salad. Enjoy!

Avocado Dressing
(makes about 1 cup)

2 medium Avocado
3-4 tsps. fresh Parsley chopped
1/2 cup Green Onion tops chopped
1/2 cup Oil or 1/4 cup Water, or
1/4 cup Lemon juice
1/8 to1/4 tsp Sea Salt
few dashes of Kelp
Cayenne-Red Pepper to taste

Blend all ingredients well & serve on salad or as dip.

Best used within 3 days.

Avocado Dressing/Dip

2 very ripe Avocados
1/2 Red Onion, chopped
1/2 Cucumber, chopped
2 Tbsp. Lime juice, squeezed

Pulse in blender until almost smooth.

Great on your favourite coleslaw, or try on your favourite green salad, or as a dip with fresh veggies.

Quick Avocado Dressing

Lemon Juice
Honey

Mix together equal amounts of the above. Mash in an avocado for a thicker dressing or dip.

Quick Caesar Dressing

Lemon Juice
Honey
1 tsp. Flax seed ground & soaked for 10 mins.

Mix these three ingredients for a Caesar or Thousand Islands-type dressing.

Tahini Dressing

1 cup raw Organic Tahini (Ground Organic Sesame Seeds)
4 Lemons or Limes, juiced
2 Cloves, chopped
Sea Salt to taste

Mix all ingredients in a bowl and put into jar for use.

Mix 2 tbsp. above mixture and you have your salad dressing. Adjust water amount for whether you want dressing or a dip.

Tarragon Dressing

2 Tbsp. minced Shallots
1 Tbsp. fresh squeezed Lemon juice
1/2 cup Olive Oil
1 Tbsp. chopped fresh Tarragon
1 tsp. Honey

Mix all ingredients & whisk well until honey is dissolved.

Poppy Seed Dressing

1/4 cup or less Honey
1 tsp. Sea Salt
1 tsp. Dry Mustard (Organic Mustard Seed Ground)
1/4 tsp. Celery seed
1/3 cup Lemon Juice
1/2 cup Flaxseed Oil
4 Tsp. Poppy seeds

In blender, combine top 5 ingredients.

While blending, gradually add oil in steady stream until thoroughly blended.
Stir in poppy seeds.

Shake well before using.

Can be used on fresh fruit as well as on your green salads.

Great Dip/ Salad Dressing

1/2 Avocado
1/2 tsp. Sea Salt
1/2 cup Parsley or Cilantro

2 large cloves Garlic
1 Lemon, juiced
1 Orange, juiced
1/4 Purple Onion

Blend everything in blender except juices and onion. Add juice in slowly, just enough juice to have blender work.
It will be very thick at first, so you will need to pulse your blender & push down with wooden spoon to keep it blending.
Finally stir in juice and onion.

Remember…less juice for thick dip, more Juice for thick or thin salad dressing.

Great substitute for "Ranch Dressing" on salads. Can also be made with zucchini, cauliflower and bell peppers. Great for pot luck suppers with raw veggies too.

Creamy Dressing

Blend:
14 ozs. soft Almond Cheese
2 Tbsp. Lemon juice
2 Tbsp. Olive Oil
2 Tbsp. Dry Mustard, (Organic Mustard Seed Ground) or Basil
Sea Salt to taste

Blend well, and use as salad dressing or dip.

Lemon Dressing

Whisk together:
1/4 cup Lemon juice
1/4 cup Olive Oil

1 tsp. fresh Garlic, minced
1/4 tsp. White Pepper

Whisk well and use on baby greens or spinach salad.

Mango Dressing

Puree peeled *Mango in blender with:
1/4 cup Lemon Juice
1 Tbsp. Unpasteurized Honey

Blend until smooth & creamy.

Delicious on baby greens or Spinach salad. Use up on same day as made

*May use any ripe soft fruit for this dressing

Red Pepper Dressing

(about 2 cups)

Puree 4 peeled, seeded red peppers

Add:
2 tbsp. Olive oil
1 Tbsp. Lemon Juice
1/4 tsp. Sea Salt
1/8 tsp. White pepper

Mix thoroughly before using.

Simple Avocado Orange Dressing

Mash ripe Avocado until soft & creamy.
Squeeze juice of 1 Orange into this and mix well. Use on green salads or cabbage salads. Also makes a great dip for veggie platter.

Easy
Entrees

Stuffed Yellow Pepper

1/2 Yellow Bell Pepper for each serving
1/4 cup Spinach chopped
1 Green Onion, chopped
Some Celery, chopped
Alfalfa Sprouts
Olive Oil
Sea Salt

Clean yellow pepper by taking out the seeds. Mix the, onion, celery, alfalfa sprouts, olive oil and sea salt.

Stuff pepper & serve.

Stuffed Red Peppers

4 firm, Red Peppers
11/4 tsp. Olive Oil
3/4 cup diced Onion
1/4 cup diced Carrot
11/2 tsp. Curry powder
2 cups baby Spinach
1/3 cup Raisins
1/3 cup chopped Walnuts

3/4 tsp. Sea Salt

Combine all above ingredients except Red Peppers. Mix well.

Cut Red Peppers in half crosswise and scoop out pulp.

Fill each half with combined ingredients.
Serve on lettuce leaf.

Cream Stuffed Red Peppers

Small Red Pepper halves, washed & seeded
Almond Sour Cream
Green onions, chopped
Parsley, chopped

Fill Red Pepper halves with Almond Sour Cream with green onions mixed into it.
Garnish with chopped parsley and serve as a great appetizer.

Sunflower Wraps

1 Red Pepper chopped
1/2 cups Sunflower Seeds, soaked,
sprouted, 1 day
juice of 1 Lemon
1 tsp. Dulse flakes
1 small Zucchini, diced
1/4 cup Scallions, diced
Broad leaf Lettuce leaves

Put Red Pepper in blender & liquefy.

Add sunflower sprouts, lemon juice and dulse flakes. Blend until smooth.

Pour mixture into bowl and add other ingredients. Mix lightly.

Spoon mixture into leaves, roll up and serve.

Pumpkin or Sunflower Herb Pate

2 cups Pumpkin or Sunflower Seeds soaked 2 hours to overnight
1/2 cup fresh Basil leaves any other fresh or dried herb of your
choice, (Sage, Savory, Thyme or Rosemary)
1 tbsp. Ground Organic Sesame Seeds
1 Lemon juiced
pinch Sea Salt
pinch of Cayenne powder
2 tbsp. Flax Oil or Olive Oil
1 clove Garlic (optional)
1 tsp. grated Ginger (optional)

Grind all ingredients in food processor until chopped.

Wrap in lettuce leaf, or nori sheets, or thin with additional liquid
and use as a dip.

Vegetable Sushi

1 cup Zucchini, riced
1/2 cup Walnuts
1/3 cup Celery
1/4 c. Green Onion diced
1/2 tsp. Sea Salt
1/8 cup Olive Oil
1/4 cup Lemon juice
1/2 tsp. Curry powder
1-2 Garlic cloves, pressed

Mix all ingredients in food processor, until fairly smooth.

Add zucchini last.

Put into Nori sheet by the spoonfuls, and spread to 1/2"-1" from edge of sheet.

Add thinly sliced Avocado, Carrot, Red Pepper, or any other veggie you would prefer. Roll up into roll, let sit for about 10 minutes. Slice in 1-2" bite size sushi rolls.

Serve with mock sour cream or dipping
Sauce, on the side.

Spaghetti Royale
(serves 7)

Shred or julienne Zucchini to create thin noodle-like strands by shredding length wise so it looks like spaghetti.

Add to spaghetti strands:
1 cup Spinach, washed, dried & rolled up & sliced into long strands. This is done by rolling the Spinach into a tight ball before slicing.

Red Pepper Basil Sauce:

2 cups fresh, diced, seeded Red Peppers
Set aside for later

Combine following ingredients and blend until moderately smooth:
2-4 cloves Garlic
3/4 cup fresh Basil, chopped
1 Lemon, juiced, or Lime, to taste
2 Tbsp. Olive Oil
4 Dates, or 1/2 cup Raisins

1 cup Sun-dried Red Peppers, soaked for 20 minutes 9 (optional)
Freshly ground White Pepper

Add this mixture to your put aside diced
Red Pepper, by hand, to make a nice looking sauce.
You may want to add some paprika at this time, or you may put
it in the sauce.

Serve Red Pepper Sauce over spaghetti on dish. Garnish with
fresh parsley.

Mock Salmon Pate

2 cups Almonds, soaked overnight
1 cup Celery, finally chopped (about 4 stalks)
1/2 cup Green Onions, chopped
1/4 cup purified Water
2 med. or large Carrots
3 tsp. Lemon juice
finely chopped whole Dulse leaf
1 head Romaine Lettuce
small handful of Parsley sprigs
3 Bell Peppers (optional)

Drain almonds and put through a food processor, to make a
smooth pate. Mix all ingredients except the lettuce or bell peppers
together in a bowl, adding the dulse to flavour. Form the mixture
into a rounded (or other shape) loaf and garnish with parsley.

Spoon onto lettuce leaves, and roll them up sushi style, fill bell
peppers, or put in Nori sheets and make sushi with julienned
vegetables.

You can serve with Almond Sour Cream, A Dip, or Dipping
Sauce.

Nutty Burger

Grind 1 lb. of your favourite nuts in a food processor. Set aside.

Combine the following ingredients and put through food processor.

1 lb. Carrots
1 medium Onion
1 tbsp. sweetener (Honey, very ripe
Banana, Raisins)
1 tbsp. Olive Oil
1-2 tsps. Poultry seasoning (or other seasoning)
Sea Salt to taste
1 clove Garlic

Add mixture to nuts that were put aside.
If the mixture is not firm enough, add some Psyllium hulls.

Form into balls, cutlets or fillets and sprinkle with a little paprika before serving.

Note: If you want "fish burgers" add seaweed (dulse, kelp, and nori) to the mixture.

Serve as loaf, burger patties, spread for crackers, or thin with some water & use as a dip.

Serves 10.

Nut Sushi

1 cup of any combination of Nuts or seeds
(Almonds, Pecans, Pine Nuts, Sunflower Seeds, Pumpkin Seeds, Walnuts, Brazil Nuts, Hazelnuts)

Raw Nori sheets
1/4 cup Cilantro
1 Avocado
1 Red Pepper
2 cloves Garlic
Sea Salt to taste

Grind nuts in food processor, mix in avocado, cilantro, red pepper, and garlic. Wrap in Nori sheets. Let sit for about 10 minutes & slice to size wanted.

Serve with Dipping sauce or Almond Sour Cream.

Nutty Loaf

2 cups Nuts or Seeds of any combination:
Almonds, Pecans, Brazil Nuts, Pine Nuts, Sunflower Seeds, Pumpkin Seeds, Walnuts, or Hazelnuts

1 Red Bell Pepper
2 cloves Garlic
1/2 Onion
1/2 Cup Zucchini
2 Tbsp. whole Pine Nuts

Grind nuts in food processor. Add vegetables and blend until smooth in food processor. Form into a loaf.

Spread Tahini Sauce (recipe follows), over the top of the loaf.

Tahini Sauce

2 Tbsp. raw Tahini (Organic Sesame Seeds Ground)
1/2 Lemon, juiced
1 tsp. Honey

2 cloves Garlic, pressed

Mix all ingredients together in blender, spread on top of loaf and decorate with pine nuts before serving.

Herbal Pizza Crust

21/2 cups Buckwheat Groats, soaked 6 hrs, sprouted 24 hours
1/3 cup Olive Oil,
3-4 Tbsp. favourite Spice
(Garlic, Indian spice Mix, Coriander, Caraway, Fennel, Oregano, etc)
1/2-1 tsp. Sea Salt or to taste
2 Tbsp. Sunflower Meal (grinding sunflower seeds in grinder until broken up)
1 cup chopped Red Pepper

Mix all ingredients in food processor, grinding groats first. Add rest of ingredients when ground, and process until a dough is formed.

Make into 7"-8" rounds about a quarter inch thick. Put into dehydrator and dry until they are dried all the way through. Turn rounds 2 or 3 times to dry evenly.
Makes 4 or 5 rounds.

Use a Red Pepper Sauce base (see page 213) or for a change use Guacamole (see page 253) as your base.
Top with your favourite vegetables.

Zesty Carrot Cups

2 cups very finely grated Carrot
1 tsp. grated Lemon zest
4 Lemon halves, after juicing

1 tsp. Unoasteurized Honey
1 Tbsp. Lemon juice or to taste
1 tsp. Olive Oil

Grate carrots until very fine. Mix Together lemon juice, zest and oil in bowl. Add Honey if too strong. Toss with carrots and fill the lemon halves with the mixture. May be served with Mock Hamburgers (see page 216) & salad.
Serves 4.

Beet Mounds

1 cup grated Beets
2 tsp. grated Ginger
1 Tbsp. Green Onion
1 sp. Lemon juice

Grate beets very fine and toss with lemon juice, green onion & grated ginger in a bowl. Add some honey if mixture is too strong. Let sit for a few minutes to let the flavours meld.

Pile on plate in mounds and top with alfalfa sprouts. Garnish & serve.

Serves 4.

Vegetable Pizza

Peel & Slice an eggplant into half-inch thick rounds.

Put in dehydrator & dry for about 1-2 hours until softened some.

Remove & add sauce:
1/2 cup dried red peppers or fresh
2-3 Tbsp. Olive Oil

1 clove Garlic, pressed
1/4 cup fresh Basil, chopped
2-4 Dates

Pour red peppers in blender with the Olive oil and pressed garlic & puree.

Add the dates and basil and blend until creamy.

Spread the sauce on the top of the dried eggplant

Just before serving add toppings of your choice, such as:

1 sliced Avocado
1 cup Yellow Squash, grated
1/2 cup Carrot, grated
1 Tbsp. fresh Parsley, chopped

You can also use Black Olives, Onion slices, Parsley, Mushrooms, or any other toppings you like. You may also return to dehydrator for 10 minutes to heat before serving.

Very good cold or warm.

Instead of Potatoes

1 Cauliflower Head, broken into florets
Water
Sea Salt
White Pepper or Peppercorns
Basil or Green onions Chopped

Put cauliflower into food processor and blend until very smooth, use very little water. Just enough as needed to keep mixture processing.

Add Sea Salt & White Pepper to taste and serve with your other recipes as mashed potatoes.

Bonnie Burritos

2 Jalapeno Peppers diced small
10 Lettuce Leaves
2 Avocados-mashed
4 Red Peppers diced
1 Orange

Mash Avocado, and mix with the peppers & Red Peppers in a bowl, Squeeze in the orange juice. Place avocado mix into the lettuce leaves and roll up cabbage roll fashion. Good idea to remove the jalapeno peppers if you are using this recipe for children.

Decadent Desserts

Fruit Pie or Cake

Crust:
Combine the following ingredients in large bowl,
mixing well:

1 cup ground Nuts, any combination
1 Tbsp. Olive Oil
1Tbsp. Honey or Dates, cut up

Topping:
Blend in a bowl the following ingredients well:
1/2 cup fresh or frozen Fruit
1/2 cup Nuts (white look nice)
1/2 cup Olive Oil
2-3 Tbsp. Honey
juice of 1 medium Lemon
1 Vanillas Bean

If needed. add water one teaspoon at a time to achieve desired
consistency.
Spread evenly over the crust.

Decorate with fruits, berries and white nuts. Chill & Serve

Tasty Pecan Apple Pie

Filling:
8 medium Apples
1/2 Tbsp. Cinnamon
1/2 tsp. Nutmeg

Crust:
11/3 cups raw Walnuts & Pecans
1/3 cup dried shredded Coconut
12 large Dates
1/2 cup Raisins, soaked
1/2 cup Pecans, soaked

Process crust ingredients in food processor by grinding together nuts & coconut, then add dates.

Mix until they form a soft ball. Not too wet.

Mold in pie plate and put aside.

In food processor, shred 4 peeled apples. Put aside.

Process the other 4 apples and add spices.

Stir in other apples that were put aside, into this apple mixture, by hand.

Pile the mixture into the pie crust.
Garnish with soaked raisins and pecans or sprinkle on some dried shredded coconut.

Serve with ice cream made from your favourite fruit. I enjoy banana on it.
Frozen Fruit Ice Cream (recipe following) is very good with this pie.

Frozen Ice Fruit (or Ice Cream)

When fruit is very ripe, cut into pieces, put in freezer bag, and freeze. Overnight is fine. up to a maximum of a week.

Remove fruit needed from freezer and let sit at room temperature for a while to let the frost start to come out. There should be still ice crystals in the fruit when you are ready to use it.

Put partially frozen fruit in blender & pulse until the texture of soft ice cream. Voila!
Ready to eat.

Put in serving dishes and top with fresh fruit or anything of your choice. Use on your favourite pie recipe, or add carob-chocolate topping. You can use pretty well all kinds of fruit for this process successfully. The result is an ice cream, better than anything you have tasted, a natural fresh fruit goody, and way better than processed ice cream Use watery fruits to make fruitsicles.

Devilish Date Cake

Crust:
2 cups mixed nuts ground lightly
(Walnuts, Almonds, Filberts, Hazelnuts, or any combination there of.)

1 cup Buckwheat Groats Flour, (grind Buckwheat Groats in coffee or nut grinder until fine)
   2 Tbsp. Honey
dash of Cinnamon

Mix above ingredients by hand to just moisten, to form into a ball.

Flatten out half of mixture on flat plate or pie plate.

Filling:
11/2–2 cups pitted Dates, soaked 30-45 minutes.
juice of 1 large Lemon zest of large Lemon (zest lemon before juicing)
3 Tbsp. Water

Put filling ingredients in blender & puree until smooth.
Spoon over flattened pie crust. Add remaining crust mixture on top.

Smooth down & press gently to firm up.

You may pop in dehydrator for 10 minutes to set.

Keep in cool place.

Enjoy.

Lemon Cream Pie

1 Tbsp. raw Honey, or 3-4 Dates
3 Tbsp. dry, shredded Coconut
1/4 Lemon, juiced
1 tbsp. Flax seed
1 Banana, mashed
1 Banana cut up

Mix all the above together and enjoy.

Apple Pie

Crust:
Make crust with soaked Almonds, or ground Hazelnuts, Filberts, or Walnuts.

Add:

3or 4 Dates

2 tbsp. Olive Oil or enough to make nuts into a ball.

Filling:

2 Apples

1/2 tsp. Cinnamon

1 tbsp. Flax oil

dash of Sea Salt

meat from young Coconut

Mix crust ingredients together in food processor, until forms into ball. Spread half of above mixture on flat plate and smooth out.

Mix filling ingredients together and spoon on top of crust on plate, spread evenly

Add remaining crust to top of filling, smooth out, and press down until even & smooth. Can serve with Almond Whipped Cream, or Frozen Fruit Ice Cream.

Delectable Fruit Salad

1 Avocado

2 Bananas

1 Mango

Chop, mix and enjoy.

Serve with Almond Whipped Cream.

Strawberry Dessert

Base:

1/2 cup Raw Almonds

6 Dates

1 tsp. Cinnamon

Chop all ingredients in food processor until it is quite soft and malleable.

Line a pie plate or dessert bowl with this base spread out line a crust.
Filling:
In blender add:
6 Strawberries
2 Bananas
1/2 cup Orange juice
1/2 cup raw Pecans

Use quantities of your choice, just make as thick and creamy as you can. It will be a creamy pink colour. Pour this mixture into the crust to fill. Garnish with sliced strawberries.

Carob Chocolate Cake

Crust:
Combine the following ingredients, in food processor mixing well.

1 cup ground Nuts
1Tbsp. Olive Oil
1cup Raisins
1 cup Raw Carob Powder
1 Vanilla Bean
1/2 tsp. Nutmeg
peel from 4 Tangerines

Form above into 1 inch layer of crust on a flat plate, keeping 1/2 for top layer of crust, or make as many layers as you like.
Filling:
1 cup Prunes soaked for 1-2 hours

Spread ground prunes between layers of crust.

Topping:

Blend the following ingredients well:

1 cup ripe Avocado
1 tsp. Olive Oil
3 Tbsp. Honey
juice of 1 medium Lemon
1 Vanilla Bean
4-5 Tbsp. Raw Carob Powder

If needed. add water one teaspoon at a time to achieve spreading consistency.

Spread evenly over the top crust, or squeeze using decorating bag. Decorate with fruits and nuts.

Chill, serve, enjoy.

Cheesecake Supreme

Pulp from Almond Milk, about 2-3 cups
Strawberries, Blueberries, etc, about 2-3 cups
1/2-1 cup honey, or 2-3 Tbsp.
Maple Syrup, or to taste
Sliced Almonds

In bowl or pan of your choice, line with cheese cloth.

Cover the bottom with the sliced Almonds.

Next, a layer of berries (approximately one third of your total berries) followed by a one inch layer of the Almond Pulp.

Continue to layer as follows:

Berries,
Drizzle of Maple Syrup or Honey over the berries,
Almond Pulp.

Keep doing this until all ingredients are gone, making sure the Almond Pulp is the final layer.

Place a flat plate over the final layer.

Gently turn over until plate is on the bottom and gently tap on upturned bowl to loosen cheesecake from bowl or pan.

Gently remove the cheesecloth and Voila, you have your cheesecake.

Enjoy!

Must
Miscellaneous

Raw Cranberry Relish

(based on recipe by Sandy Cook)

2 cups fresh Cranberries
1 whole fresh Orange

1 cup Walnuts or Hazelnuts
1/2 cup Honey or Dates or Raisins

Wash orange very well and chop into small pieces.

Combine with the rest of the ingredients and blend in food processor until well blended.

Serve with garden burger, nut loaf or in a wrap as a festive treat.

Better Than Butter

2 lemons, juiced
2 Tbsp. Olive Oil
1/4 cup water
1/2 cup pine nuts
1 tsp. sea salt
1/2 cup Coconut Butter/Oil

Blend all ingredients until smooth, adding more water if needed.

Add 1/2 cup Coconut butter, fresh, or purchased at health food store. Blend in very well.

Pour into container & chill well in refrigerator.

Gazpacho

In bowl combine:

2 cups chopped Red Peppers
1/2 cup chopped Cucumber
1/2 cup chopped Celery
1/2 cup Red Pepper, chopped
3 Tbsp. chopped Cilantro
1 tsp. Sea Salt to taste

Blend half of this mixture with 1/4 cup
Tomato Dressing (see page 202).
Process until smooth.

Top with 2 Tbsp. Avocado Dressing
(See page 195)

Sprinkle with 2 Tbsp. Raw pumpkin seeds.

Indian Spice Mix

8 tsp. dry Mustard
4 tsp. ground Fenugreek
4 tsp. ground Cumin
2 tsp. ground Turmeric
2 tsp. ground Ginger
2 tsp. ground Coriander
2 tsp. ground Cloves
1/2 tsp. ground Cinnamon

In small bowl combine all above ingredients. Mix well to blend.
Pour into air-tight glass jar and store in dark cupboard or fridge to
preserve flavour.

Can be used in mock hamburger or sprinkled on fresh vegetables, or in salad dressings.

Seasoned Sunflower Seeds

2 cups raw Sunflower seeds, soaked
6 hours. Sprouted one day.
2 Tbsp. Lemon Juice
1 tsp. Onion juice, squeezed
1/8 tsp. Garlic, squeezed
1/8 tsp. Cayenne Powder

Put sunflower seeds in bowl and cover with 3-4 times the amount of water, than you have seeds. Cover with cloth and let soak overnight.

Rinse thoroughly, put sunflower seeds in Sprouting bag, cover with cloth and let sprout for 1 day. Rinse twice during the day.

Next day, rinse and dry sunflower seeds on a clean towel. Place in bowl and add rest of ingredients, mixing well.

Spread seeds on dehydrator sheet, allowing space between them and dehydrate for 8 to 12 hours.

Store in Refrigerator

Organic Live Raw Sauerkraut
(Read Before Making)

Save 2 clean cabbage leaves and put aside for later

Cut cabbage in quarters

Remove core from these quarters and discard

Slice very thinly or shred 1ˢᵗ quarter until it is the texture you like
Put this into a large crock type bowl
Add 1 tsp. Celtic Sea Salt
Squeeze this mixture with your hands until it becomes wet

Do 2ⁿᵈ quarter by shredding or slicing
Add to crock like bowl with 1ˢᵗ quarter
Add 1 tsp. Celtic Sea Salt.
Squeeze with hands until it becomes wet

Do 3ʳᵈ. quarter by slicing or shredding and adding to 1ˢᵗ & 2ⁿᵈ quarters already in bowl.
Add 1 tsp. Celtic Sea Salt.
Squeeze with hands until wet

Do 4ᵗʰ or last quarter by shredding or slicing and adding to others in bowl
Add 1 tsp. Celtic Sea Salt
Squeeze with hands until wet

Add 1/2 —1 cup of water to bowl after cabbage(Some cabbages are very dry)(Helps to culture)

Clear sides of bowl until clean. Add 2 leaves saved at beginning, by placing over top of the shredded cabbage in bowl.

Place flat saucer or plate on top of cabbage leaves in bowl. (Just smaller than bowl)

Put weight (Large jar of water is good) on top of saucer in bowl

Cover with a large cloth to keep out dust and bugs

Set aside to Kraut for 4 or 5 days(Culturing)

When kraut is done (after 4or 5 days) open up and check to see if it is as you like it. If not let set longer. Taste Test
Check to see there are no brown or black cabbage in bowl. If there is remove it and discard it before mixing the Kraut up. This is wayward bacteria that formed in the pot and you DO NOT want TO EAT IT? Hasn't hurt the Kraut.

Put new Kraut in glass jars and store in refrigerator as you use it. Will keep for about a month

Salsa Cruda

4 large cloves Garlic
1 cup chopped Cilantro
1 bunch of Scallions, 8-10 white parts
1 sweet bell Pepper, Red, Yellow, Orange or Purple
1 Jalapeno Pepper, chopped, seeds removed
4 large, ripe Red Peppers
1Tbsp. fresh, minced Oregano Leaves
1/2 tsp. Sea Salt

Pulse all ingredients in food processor until coarsely chopped, or to a large sized mince.

The sauce should be lumpy and all ingredients recognizable.

May be used on Spaghetti Royale or on top of your Pizza as Red Pepper Sauce.

Guacamole

2 Avocados
1 Lemon, juiced
1Red Pepper
1/2 tsp. Mexican Spice

Cumin, or Cilantro, to taste

In food processor, blend lemon juice with half of red pepper and half of avocados. Chop until fairly chunky.

Finely dice the other half red pepper.
Mash remaining avocado, leaving it chunky also.

Combine both mixtures and season with the Mexican Spice, cumin or Cilantro and additional lemon juice if needed, or to taste.

May be used for base of Pizzas.

Mexican Spice Mix

Chili Peppers
Dehydrated Garlic
Dehydrated Onion
Paprika
Cumin
Celery Seed
Dehydrated Oregano
Dehydrated Red Pepper
Ground Bay Leaf

Mix all ingredients well and store in tightly sealed glass jar, in dark cupboard or fridge to preserve flavour.

Use in your Mexican Dishes, Pates and Salad Dressings.

Veggie, Cheese Snacks
1/2 Red, Orange, or Purple Bell Pepper
1—2 Inch Green or Red Cabbage Leaf
3-4 Celery Sticks

Turnip Or Rutabaga

Slice the above ingredients to look like chips.

Make a cheese spread by soaking 1-2 cups almonds overnight
In morning, blanche quickly & skin.

Put in blender & add 1-2 cups water, just enough to keep blender
working.

Pour in plate & dehydrate for 6-8 hours, or until it has a cream
cheese consistency.

Serve on platter surrounded by chips.

Date Treat

Your Choice of Dates—Usually 10-12
Same amount of Almonds-10-12

Take pits out from center of dates, if they have them, or purchase
pitted dates.

Put almonds in centers and enjoy as a snack treat.

In
Conclusion

This brings me to the end of this book that I dearly hope will be able to help you to understand and make the transition from cooked food to the raw food life-style, if you choose to do so. I hope that I have included everything to make your transition easier by not having to go out and buy fifteen books to be able to get started on your new decision.

I trust the explanations on the major factors controlling your health (Cooked Food, Live Enzymes, Water, Oils, Fats and Supplements) have given you an insight into these issues that could affect the way your body is acting & help you to be able to integrate the information into your new lifestyle.

The contents of this book have been written and the explanations brought to you, to have you understand why it is that raw food is so important to our well being.

The diseases that are rampant, could well be addresses by looking at why they are so prevalent today. Try to make changes to yourselves, if only to fight these disease from where they originate. The body and what we put into it.

Get a buddy to raw food with. It will make it easier for you to stay on track. Do this for at least 2 months; as that is the time frame for the temptations to be the strongest for you. Remember that cooked food diet is an addiction, and we must train our minds to overlook the habits we have and to create new habits.

It isn't hard, but we must be persistent. Here are the things that may take you back to the cooked food trap. Please be aware of them, and be prepared to substitute them with raw food or have a plan of recourse, so you don't submit to them.

They are:
hunger,
anger,
disappointment,
loneliness,
tired, etc.

Listen to your body and know what the signs are.
I wish you all a happy transition, and if you need more information or support in your new venture, please feel free to go to my webpage and ask me the questions or concerns you may have.

The webpage is: http://www.liverawkitchebn.com

Appendix A: Menu Suggestions

The All Raw Diet Menu Suggestions

Do feel free to eat large quantities of fruits and vegetables if you would like to. You should feel free to eat an abundance of food if your body desires it. As time passes you will eat less and less as your food is assimilated better and your body does not require as much food.

You should remember that physical exercise goes along with any good diet program. The Raw Nutrition you are taking in is coupled with physical motion, for the body to operate at its peek.

These recipes are guidelines only, to get you started on your All-Raw Diet for better health. I also eat in this way to satiate my hunger.

This is a great diet to help the transition from cooked foods to raw foods, as the fats in it will fill you up and satisfy your hunger pangs. The important thing is to feed your body what it needs to have and you will not have a problem with the transition from cooked foods. Remember to have exercise daily and keep your body active. This benefits your body and your transition.

All foods mentioned are considered to be ORGANIC grown foods.

Day 1-Monday:

Morning:

2 lbs, Watermelon, (not seedless), Juiced
Afternoon:

One large Lettuce, Cucumber, Red Pepper, and Green Onion salad with one handful of Raw Sunflower Seeds, 1 Avocados, and 1/2 a fresh squeezed Lemon.

Evening:

1 Nectarine
1 stick of Celery
1/2 Avocado
Juiced
Snack:

1or 2 Nectarines

Day 2-Tuesday:

Morning:

1/2 large Honeydew Melon
The water from 1 Coconuts
Juiced

Afternoon:

2 Oranges
1 Small green-leafed salad, containing at least 1 ribs of Celery, 10-20 Walnuts ground and fresh squeezed Lemon Juice as dressing.

Snack:

2 Oranges, juiced

Evening:

Large Salad containing 80% green-leafed Vegetables, 1 Avocados and an Orange Juice squeezed dressing.
1 pint of freshly made Vegetable juice containing at least 60% green Vegetables, 40% other vegetables or fruits (i.e. Apple, Cucumber, etc)

Day 3-Wednesday

Morning:

2Apples
5-10 Pecans or Macadamia Nuts with Lettuce, juiced

Afternoon:

Cucumber, Red Pepper, Zucchini mixed salad. Squeezed Orange as dressing.

Snack:

1 Apples
Assorted Greens (Green Cabbage, Lettuce, Endive, etc)

Evening:

Large salad containing 80% green-leafed Vegetables including Kale or Spinach eaten with 1 Nectarine chopped and an Orange squeezed as dressing.

Day 4-Thursday

Morning:

1/2pint freshly made
Grapefruit juice

Afternoon:

2 bowls of Berries (Strawberries, Blueberries, etc.)
1 small Lettuce salad with Cucumber
1 Avocado and 10-15 Almonds ground
Lemon juice & Olive oil as dressing

Snack:

2 Nectarines

Evening:

Large salad containing 80% green-leafed Vegetables, and an Orange squeezed as dressing. Add several servings of raw Dulse Seaweed to the salad if desired.

Day 5-Friday

Morning:

2-Oranges (eat the white pith too)
10-Macadamia Nuts ground with Lettuce

Afternoon:

Cucumber, Red Pepper, Green Onion & Zucchini mixed Salad.
Add Extra Virgin Olive Oil and squeezed Lemon as Dressing

Snack:

2 Oranges
Assorted Greens (Spinach, Baby Bok Choy, Endive), juiced

Evening:

Large Salad containing 80% green-leafed Vegetables,
1 Avocados, and an Orange squeezed as dressing.
1 pint freshly made Vegetable juice containing at least 60% green
Vegetables, 40% other Vegetables or Fruits (i.e. Pear, Zucchini,
Asparagus, etc.)

Day 6-Saturday

Morning:

20-30 Berries (Strawberry, Blueberry, etc)
mixed with lettuce or mixed with 1 Avocado

Afternoon:

1/2 Cantaloupe
1 pint of freshly made Vegetable juice containing at least 50%
green Vegetables, 50% Apples, or Pears

Snack:

1 Handful of Sunflower Seeds

Evening:

Large salad containing 80% green Vegetables including 2 ribs
Celery, 1 Avocados, and Extra Virgin Olive Oil & Lemon Juice as
dressing. Add several servings of Raw Dulse Seaweed and Raw
grated Garlic to the salad if desired.

Day 7-Sunday

Morning:

No Breakfast

Afternoon:

Large salad containing 80% green-leafed Vegetables, 1 Avocado, Dulse Seaweed, and an Orange blended with Raw, Organic Flax Seed Oil

Snack:

1 Apple
2 ribs of Celery
Evening:

The water of 1 Coconut 1 pint freshly made Vegetable juice containing at least 60% green Vegetables, 40% other Vegetables or Fruits (1 each Asian Pear, Broccoli, Cauliflower, etc.)

Appendix B: Glossary

Addiction:
a condition in which we find ourselves, upon indulging in a habit for a long time and it becomes very, very difficult to break. (i.e. smoking, alcoholism, chocolate addiction, cooked food addiction, coffee addiction, etc)

Caffeine:
component of some products that stimulate the nervous system, and destroys the enzymes in your body. Also may cause dehydration. Cooked Food: food that has been heated over 105 degrees to be cooked. This causes the nutrition to be destroyed. No food value for your body, and it takes 24 hours to be pushed through the system.

Colon:
main organ of the body that feeds nutrition to your organs and glands and is responsible for removing the waste and toxins from your body. When working well, it moves wastes 2 to 3 times a day. Any less it is impaired.

Craving:
the urge to need to consume a certain food at a given time. Some cravings are so bad, that we would do anything to get our hands on the thing we are craving (this is an addiction).This usually is the result of a toxin in our body wanting the food, yeast, etc. to feed it, and allow it to grow, and/or stay alive in our body. No toxic food, it dies and goes away.

Detoxify:
removing the toxins from our body, in a controlled manner, mostly. Eliminating the excess acids & chemicals we have acquired over the years. This is accumulated from our environment, the food we eat, the water we drink, pesticides, herbicides, etc. that welcome in contact with, every day of our lives.

Enzymes:
"sparks" of life to your body. If no enzymes your body, you die. Acquired through foods that are alive. Only in raw, natural foods. Like leafy green vegetables, etc. Your body does not use the synthetic enzymes found in supplements.

Fasting:
just not eating, though people do drink juices & water during their fast period. Can run from one day to two weeks. Great for helping the body to cleanse.

Fever:
is the body raising your temperature to a high level to try and eradicate toxins from your body. It is not dangerous. Should be left to run course. Usually only 24-36 hours Using something to stop it, will divert the body from ridding you of toxins, to getting rid of the chemical you just gave it. Allow the body to chase the toxins out. Assist it by resting & drinking lots of water.

Fluoride:
a chemical used for treating city water system, to protect the enamel on your teeth. Also used in toothpaste, etc for tooth protection. Now found to be very dangerous to the body.*

Ingredients:
contents of products you use. Must read labels to find what you are buying. These have to be listed on the products you are purchasing,

though some may not be required to be listed. Sometimes, not. Read, read, read. Be careful of the words, "natural" and "organic." Read, read, and make sure you are getting what you want. As natural as possible.

Juicing:
breaking down the fresh produce into juice by a using a machine that extracts the juice from the pulp. Very good for you, as the body uses it instantly, and the good nutrition soars through your body like small jets. Particularly useful for chronic disease repair.

Mucus:
a phlegm type of liquid that we usually first notice in the throat. We have to clear our throats, usually quite often after eating something sweet, or dairy products. This mucus is built up over time, as it forms in our stomach to protect us from poison (cooked food).Once its job is done, it stores itself in the bottom of the lungs, awaiting removal from the body through activity.

Nutrients:
array of vitamins & minerals, enzymes, etc, that our bodies need each and every day, for us to be able to live our lives. Without them, the spark goes out & we die. Derived from natural, raw fruits, vegetables, seeds& nuts.

Oils:
good-means the oils the body can use and are a benefit to the body. Like, Olive Oil, Flaxseed Oil, Sesame Seed Oil, etc. bad-oils your body cannot use or assimilate, and just clogs your systems. Like, Canola Oil, Safflower Oil, Vegetable Oil (canola) Lard, etc. Most shelf
dressings have these oils in them. Check your labels.

Organic:
foods grown under pure, controlled conditions, with no chemicals or pesticides, herbicides, etc. Soils are kept re-nourished with natural soil enhancers. No DNA changed seed used. Full of natural nutrients.

Raw food:
food that is uncooked in any way. May be dried under 110 degrees. Fresh fruits, vegetables, seeds, nuts, etc. Foods that can be digested and used by the body for optimum nutrition. Full of natural nutrients, enzymes, etc.

Sprouting:
soaking seeds, nuts of all kinds and allowing them to begin to grow into sprouts. These sprouts are very rich in enzymes and nutrients at this stage of their new growth. Very good in raw food recipes and very easy to sprout. Just need large jars & seeds, nuts, etc.

Supplements:
replacing natural nutrients with synthetic formed vitamins, minerals, etc. The body cannot use these synthetics, so they pass through the system without dong you any good. Just very expensive urine. Found on most health food, drugstore, & nutrition store shelves. Know what you are buying.

Temptations:
something that is put in front of you that you may be trying to omit from your lifestyle. i.e. Your favourite cooked food, when you are trying to eliminate it from your habits. Cigarettes, when you are trying to quit smoking. These temptations need a diversion, when they come along. One diversion is to have something raw instead, ie, sunflower seeds, raw carrot sticks, banana, etc. These temptations will go away, once we control them.

Appendix C:
Acid/Alkaline Chart

We need to have the correct balance between alkaline and acid in our systems, to be healthy. A diet of 80% alkaline and 20% acid forming foods will keep a healthy, balanced system. Raw food is best.

Eliminating all acid foods from your diet to begin with, will help you greatly in getting back to your acid/ alkaline balance in your body. It allows the excess acid to be cleaned from your system without having more added to it.

You can then re-introduce more acid foods back into your body to keep you balanced.

Here is a list of some of the foods that are acid, alkaline and neutral. This will help you to distinguish which ones are acid and which are alkaline and what ones are neutral. It is okay to eat the alkaline foods and the neutral food groups when you are initially cleaning your body and getting it back into balance.

Because of the speed at which our digestive system works on different food groups, it is important to remember to always eat the fruits by themselves. Fruit digests very quickly. Avoid eating fruit with the nut food group.

Acid	Neutral	Alkaline
All antibiotics	almonds	almonds
All fried foods	apples	blackberries
Baking soda	bananas	broccoli
Alcohol	blueberries	cantalope
Artificial sweeteners	brazil nuts	cinnamon
Beans-fresh & dried	buckwheat	coconut
Beef	cauliflower	diakon radish
Beer	carrots	endive
Brussel sprouts	chestnuts	garlic
Butter	dates	grapefruit
Carob	eggplant	honeydew melon
Casein	figs	kale
Ketchup	grapes	kolerabi
All cheeses	honey	limes
Lentils	lettuce	mangos
Chicken	millet	molasses
Mineral water	organic flax seed	oil mustard greens
All eggs	oranges	nectarines
Chickpeone	peaches	onions
Goat cheese	pears	papayas
Cocoa/chocolate	pineapple	peppers
Coffee	plums	poppy seeds
Lima beans	pumpkins	raspberry
Maple syrup	raisins	sea salt
Corn		tangerines
Corn starch		water melon
All rice yams		
Strawberry		
Cranberries		
Flour		
Jams/ jellies		
Ice cream		
All dairy milk		

Acids Continued

Lard & products
Lobster
Muscles
Peanuts
Oat bran
Hydrogenated oils
Peas
Pork
All grains
All soy beans & products
Sugars
Tomatoes
Turkey
Veal

Appendix D: Sprouting Chart

Sprouting Chart

Variety	Soak (hours)	Dry Measure*	Length at Harvest	Ready in (days)	Sprouting Tips	Nutritional Highlights	Suggested Uses
Adzuki	12	1 cup	1/2-1"	3-5	Easy sprouter. Try short and long.	high quality protein: iron, vitamin C	casserole. Oriental dishes, salads, sandwiches, sprout leaves
Alfalfa	4-6	3-4 tbsp.	1-1 1/2"	4-6	Place in light to develop chlorophyll 1-2 days before.	vitamin A, B, C, E & K; rich in minerals and trace elements	juices, salads, sandwiches, soup, sprouts loaves
Almond	12	1 cup	0"	1	Swells up, does not sprout.	rich in protein, fats, minerals, vitamins, B and E	breads, cheeses, desserts, dressings, milks
Cabbage	4-6	1/3 cup	1"	4-5	Develops chlorophyll.	vitamins A, C & U trace elements	coleslaw, salads, sandwiches soups
Chick Peas	12	1 cup	1/2"	2-3	Mix with lentils & wheat, or use alone.	carbohydrates, fiber, protein, minerals	breads, casserole, dips, salads, spreads, sprout loaves
Clover	4-6	3 tbsp.	1-1 1/2"	4-5	Mix with other seeds, Develops chlorophyll.	vitamins A & C; trace elements	breads, salads, sandwiches soups
Corn	12	1 cup	1/2"	2-3	Use sweet corn. Try short & long.	carbohydrates, fiber, minerals vitamins A, B, & E	breads, cereals, grain dishes granola, snacks
Cow Peas	12	1 cup	1/2-1"	3-6	Grow in dark. Try short & medium.	protein, vitamins A & C, minerals	Oriental dishes, salads, sprout loaves
Fenugreek	8	1/2 cup	1/2-1"	3-5	Pungent flavour, mix with other seeds.	rich in iron, phosphorus, trace elements	casseroles, curries, juices, salads, soups, sprout loaves
Green Peas	12	1 cup	1/2"	2-3	Use whole peas.	carbohydrates, fiber, protein, minerals, vitamins A & C	casseroles, dips, dressings, salads, soups, sprout loaves
Lentil	12	1 cup	1/4-3/4"	3-5	Earthy flavour. Try short & long. Versatile sprout.	rich in protein, iron and other minerals, vitamin C	breads, casseroles, curries, marinated vegetables, salads, soups, spreads, sprout loaves
Millet	8	1 cup	1/4"	2-3	Use unhulled type.	carbohydrates, fiber, vitamins B & E, protein	breads, casseroles, cereals, salads, soups

Sprouting Chart - *Continued*

Variety	Soak (hours)	Dry Measure*	Length at Harvest	Ready in (days)	Sprouting Tips	Nutritional Highlights	Suggested Uses
Mung	12	1/2 cup	1/2-1 1/2"	3-6	Grow in dark Rinse in cold water for 1 min.	high quality protein; iron, potassium, vitamin C	juices, Oriental dishes, salads, sandwiches, soups, sprout loaves
Mustard	4-6	1/4 cup	1"	4-5	Hot flavour; mix with other seeds.	mustard oil, vitamin A & C, minerals	juices, salads, sandwiches, soups
Oats	12	1 cup	1/4-1/2"	2-3	Find whole sprouting type.	vitamins B & E, protein, carbohydrates, fiber, minerals	breads, casseroles, cereals, soups, sprout loaves
Pumpkin	8	1 cup	0"	1	Swells up, does not sprout.	proteins, fats, vitamin E, phosphorus, iron, zinc	breads, cereals, cheeses, desserts, dressings, milks, snacks, sprout loaves, yogurts
Radish	4-6	1/4 cup	1"	4-5	Hot flavour; mix with other seeds. Develops chlorophyll	potassium, vitamin C	dressings, juices, Mexican style food, salads, sandwiches, soups
Rye	12	1 cup	1/4-1/2"	2-3	Try mixing with wheat and lentils	vitamins B & E, minerals, protein, carbohydrates	breads, cereals, granola, milks, salads, soups
Sesame dressings	4-6	1 cup	0"	1-2	Tiny sprout, turns bitter if left too long.	rich in protein, calcium and other minerals, vitamins B & E, fats, fiber	breads, candies, cereals, cheeses, milks, salads, yogurts
Sunflower	8	2 cups	0-1/2"	1-3	Used hulled seeds. Mix with alfalfa and grow 4-5 days.	rich in minerals, fats, proteins, vitamins B & E	breads, cereals, cheeses, desserts, dressings, milks, salads, soups, sprout loaves, yogurts
Triticale	12	1 cup	1/4-1/2"	2-3	A grain hybrid like wheat.	see wheat	see wheat
Watercress	4-6	4 tbsp.	1/2"	4-5	Spicy; mix with other seeds	vitamins A & C, minerals	breads, garnishes, salads, sandwiches
Wheat	12	1 cup	1/4-1/2"	2-3	Try short and long. For sweeter taste, mix with other seeds.	carbohydrates, protein, vitamins B & E, phosphorus	breads, cereals, desserts, granola milks, salads, snacks, soups

* per half-gallon jar   From the Book "Sprouting" by Ann Wigmore

Appendix E: Juicers

There are many kinds of **juicers** on the market today. It all depends on the job that you want to use it for. A high speed juicer is recommended to juice your hard vegetables and fruits, like carrots, beets, celery, etc. There are many kinds to choose from, some of the most important and popular are:

Centrifugal Juicer: this high speed juicer separates the juice from the pulp through a plastic or steel basket. It chops the fruits and vegetables, and spins them at high speed, leaving the pulp in the basket until discarded.

Centrifugal With Pulp Ejector: this juicer works basically the same as the one listed above, but ejects the pulp from the basket into a waiting container on the outside of the machine.

Masticating Juicer: this high speed juicer masticates the fruit or vegetable into a paste, then squeezes the juice out through a screen in the machine.

Wheat Grass Juicer: this juicer is a more heavy duty juicer than the others, and runs slower, as wheat grass is a very tough grain to break down. It doesn't masticate the fruit or vegetable, as the other high speed juicers do. It presses the juice from the produce instead of turning it into a paste or chopping it up first. You will get more beneficial juice from this machine as it retains more of the nutrients of the fruit & vegetables.

Manual Juicer: though it has no motor to help with, it is a very efficient tool. This juicer is one that usually contains two or three parts. The cap to put the juicing material into, the juicer itself, and the cup or container to catch the juice in. This entails forcing the fruit or vegetable by hand, over the juicing section to extract the juice. You can do this by grating the fruit or vegetable first and making it into a paste and putting it into a sprouting bag (can buy these at my website

http://www.liverawkitchen.com,) then put over the juicer section, and squeeze the juice from it. This gives you a very superior juice.

Some selected juicers, for comparison, are:

Vita-Mix Juicer: High-speed, heavy duty juicer that will last a long time and juice everything that you may want to juice. This machine is double duty as well. It is used as a blender, juicer, shredder, etc. Easy to Clean. Runs between $200-$500

Jack LaLannes Power Juicer: this juicer is purchased from the States. High speed and heavy duty as well. It is very powerful and extracts to a very dry pulp. Can use the whole fruit, as it has a fairly large chute. Has a large pulp catcher. It is a masticating type juicer, with ejection of pulp. Juice is pulp free & requires no straining before drinking. Easy to clean. Runs between *$200-$400.

Champion Juicer: this high speed heavy duty juicer is also ideal for everyday juicing. It is a masticating juicer with pulp ejection. This juicer can do double duty as a grinder, blender as well. Easy to clean. Runs between *$250-$400.

Wheat Grass Juicer: this juicer is heavy duty, slow speed to press all the juices out of the fruits and vegetables, slowly to retain the highest content of nutrients. This juicer can press the heavier, stronger vegetables and grasses without getting too hot. The motor will last longer and the juice will not be oxidized. Runs about *$500-$1000

Where to Purchase these Juicers

As a rule, most department or hardware stores have these juicers on hand. You must shop around to get what you are looking for. Also you may go to the webpage: www.liverawkitchen.com and get more information on them.

Health food stores and bulk food stores are also now starting to handle different types of juicers. My suggestion is, that you do your homework on what type of juicer you want, and what you want to use it for, before you go shopping for one.

You won't regret purchasing one of the most important tools you will use in your raw food lifestyle. It will become your buddy and you will be using it mostly every day. So be sure you are purchasing the one you want to use.

*Juicer prices subject to change. Used as comparisons only.

Appendix F:
End Notes

Water Contamination
Info pages at:
http://www.dep.state.fl.us/water/drinkingwater/microcon.html

Fluoride
Info pages at:
http://www.all-natural.com/f/effects.html

Dehydration
Info pages at:
http://www.dep.state.fl.us/water/drinkingwater/inorg.com.html

Caffeine
Info pages at:
http://www.mckinley.uiuc.edc/health.info/drug.alc/caffeine.html

Cooking Food
Info pages at:
http://www.news.bbc.co.uk/1/hi/health/2442845.stm

"After the Doctors…What Can You Do"
Author Ron Garner
Info at:
http://www.hopeforhealth.com

QXCI Testing

Info at:

http://www.theqxci.com

Rose Stevens, Quantum, Biofeedback

Therapist email at: rose2279@shaw

Letter from Rose Stevens R.T.,

on Elyse's QXCI Analysis

What is a QXCI analysis?

Rose Stevens is former laboratory technologist who has now applied those skills to become a dark field Microscopist and a QXCI Quantum Xxeroid Consciousness Interface Therapist.

The basis of the QXCI biofeedback analysis is the transmission of 65million tiny electromagnetic signals into the body, many times per second through sensors that are strapped around the wrists, ankles and forehead. This information is then interfaced with the program and measured against over 8000 different frequencies in the matrix. These pulses map the body and its organs and reveal anomalies within the body. It reveals if you're hydrated sufficiently or whether you need oxygen. The machine also indicates the presence of worms, fungus, viruses, bacteria and toxins. It has a heart, brain and body scan as well as dealing with issues of nutrition, vitamins and minerals.

Depending on what is found during the analysis, the QXCI can then use scalar and electromagnetic waves to rebalance the body, and specific homeopathics and herbs may be used to continue with the healing and detoxification process.

Elyse Nuff—QXCI analysis

After hooking Elyse Nuff up to the QXCI for a biofeedback analysis, **I can honestly say that I have never seen anyone with such a balanced health profile. Elyse had no pathogenic parasites, fungus, viruses or bacteria in her body. You see, her eating alive and raw has created a proper "ph" balance in her body that does not allow for the overgrowth of such organisms.**

This confirms the Dr. Bechamp and Dr. Enderlien's theory of pleomorphism. In other words, contrary to Louis Pasteur's germ theory, bugs do not cause disease. It is the unhealthy terrain that allows for the growth of these organisms.

I see many ill clients whose blood looks like a swamp, but Elyse's was as clean as a river. The levels of industrial and environmental toxins were extremely low, as she eats only organic pesticide free vegetables. Her pleomorphic panel on the QXCI (live blood cell analysis) was indicative of the "immortal blood" that Dr Bob Beck talks about with his process of "Blood Electrification." I have only seen this kind of profile with people who follow the "BECK PROTOCOL."
Even if they do clean up their blood with the Beck units, they will never maintain their healing if they do not alkalize their bodies. I believe that the simplest way we can achieve this, is through eating alive and raw.

In the nutritional panel, all vitamins and minerals were balanced and the digestion was perfect. In the anti aging program the DHEA, growth hormone, elastin, and calcium in tissues were all within normal levels. I have very rarely seen this kind of balance, either. All the chakras were balanced as well as the emotional profile.

This did not surprise me, because Elyse is well aware how much emotions contribute to our over all health, as she practices cellular emotional release techniques in her clinic. You see negative emotions can also make us acidic and throw off our ph. Not only is it important what goes into the mouth, but it is equally important as to what comes out of the mouth.

The QXCI analysis has confirmed to me that **'Eating Alive And Raw'** works!! Elyse is a dynamic living testimony of this!! I salute you Elyse for practicing what you preach!!!

Disclaimer: The QXCI does not diagnose illnesses, but rather analyzes imbalances and nutrition, and reduction of stressors are addressed within the parameters of natural health and biofeedback. A QXCI therapist is not an allopathic doctor and does not pretend to be, but is a nutritional, wellness and biofeedback specialist. Those seeking consul, advice, opinions, biofeedback or points of view and/or programs within the scope of the attending therapist, do so at their own free will.

Rose Stevens R.T
Holistic Practitioner and Quantum Therapist
Kelowna B.C, rose2279@shaw.ca

Elyse's Story

Moving from being a year away from having liver cancer and having three deteriorating discs in my lower back, to being healthy and vital again, was the biggest joy in my life. Within a very short time, I lost the unnecessary body fat that I was carrying around with me, and my body is now maintaining a natural body weight that gives me the energy and vitality I need to be young again.

In my 60's now, I feel better than I did when I was sixteen. This is all thanks to the Raw Food and live nutrition I have been giving my body. If I can do this for my health, anyone can.

Within 2 years plus my discs in my lower back rebuilt and are now solid and healthy. This is due to the natural calcium being fed into the bones by the enzymes in the live foods. This has created more bone mass and stronger bones for me. I no longer have backache or trauma there. My body is more flexible and supple as well. I now live with complete overall good health.

-Elyse

Recipe Index

Easy Entrees

Over 400% more…

Vitality, stamina and clarity. Enhanced, continuous, sustained energy, and true natural muscle mass, when living the raw food lifestyle.
THERE'S NOTHING LIKE IT FOR WEIGHT CONTROL, THE PROBLEM JUST DOSESN'T COME BACK. Frustrated with your diet plans? Try the simple method of controlling your weight, while keeping your body healthy. Diseases and health problems just melt away. This is the easy way…As Nature Intended. A healthy, vital body all your life. This book is your guide.

The QXCI analysis has confirmed to me that 'Eating Alive And Raw' works!! Elyse is a dynamic living testimony of this!! I salute you Elyse for practicing what you preach!!!
Rose Stevens R.T., Holistic Practitioner and Quantum Therapist

About the author…*Elyse Nuff S.T.C.,R.F.C.,W.H.C.*
Whol-istic Health Consultant for the past 16 years. Publisher, Poet, Certified raw Chef, Author, Coach, Trainer & Teacher, Artist and Grandmother four times over. Trained in the art of looking for the cause of a disease and healing with nature.
Spent most of her growing years in search of true health and well being. Has researched the aspect of well being outside of the traditional methods so popular over the past century.

Living the research and bringing everyone the proven experience of being there. Always alert to the methods of approaching good health. Initiated her own back to health & well being. (testimonial inside) Resides on Salt Spring Island in BC, and travels extensively, educating others in the ways of being responsible for their own health and environment.

Teaching others the art of Cellular Healing, correcting their Spinal Problems, and teaching the Raw Food Lifestyle, to those wanting to improve their health.

The author of a yearly food calendar called "Live raw Kitchen", issued every November. Elyse can be reached through her webpage:

http://www.liverawkitchen.com
liverawkitchen@gmail.com

CPSIA information can be obtained at www.ICGtesting.com
Printed in the USA
BVOW032242011112

304493BV00002B/23/P